Further praise for *Macrobiotics for Life*

"In *Macrobiotics for Life,* Simon Brown provides a non-dogmatic, holistic view of healing. From beginning to end, his conversational style allows readers to view him as a fellow traveler down life's road—a trusted friend providing gentle guidance. The sections on emotional healing provide a significant addition to macrobiotic literature and fill a long-standing void. The depth of understanding and the numerous analogies, examples, practical exercises, and useful summaries at the end of each chapter make this book a must-have for anyone interested in health and well-being."

—CARL FERRÉ, president of the George Ohsawa Macrobiotic Foundation
and author of *Pocket Guide to Macrobiotics* and *Acid and Alkaline Companion*

"Living a healthy life is quickly becoming a revolutionary act. Simon Brown's book brings practical insight and broad vision to the transformative study and practice of macrobiotics."

—BILL TARA, macrobiotic teacher and counselor

"Simon Brown brings macrobiotics into the twenty-first century. By emphasizing the mental, emotional, and spiritual areas of our life, he shows how these intersect for each of us, especially in our way of eating. By inviting you to reflect on these issues, he helps lead you to a profound level of self-discovery. He gently educates you on the key concepts of macrobiotic principles so that you will find them easy to embrace. There is no dogma of good versus bad; instead, Simon provides the tools to understand balance through your experience. This book excels by opening the door wide for lifestyle changes that will influence you, your family—especially children—and your relationships in new, exciting, and healthy ways."

—MICHAEL ROSSOFF, LAc, macrobiotic teacher, counselor,
and founder of Macrobiotics Today

"At last—a book that in a very clear and direct, simple and sincere way leads you into the depths of the macrobiotic way of life. This is 'the best of' the most precious insights and experience gained from a lifetime of macrobiotic philosophy and practice. Simon Brown has shown us the wholeness of a macrobiotic approach to life, the indisputable bond that exists between emotions, attitude, eating habits, breathing, exercising, and healing on all levels of our lives. He fills the void in literature on macrobiotics and provides an excellent compass for anyone who wants to take a healthier and happier road to a great life."

—**JADRANKA BOBAN PEJIĆ, macrobiotic teacher**
and award-winning cookbook author

"Simon Brown has created a broad and highly accessible platform by eliminating much of the conceptual dogma and rigidity that has plagued macrobiotics for so many years. He has opened a new front by examining the role that our emotional life plays in terms of overall health. To his credit, he is also unafraid to venture outside the artificial constraints of macrobiotics by citing other bodies of work that can complement one's practice. This book is equally useful for those wanting to launch their own macrobiotic practice and more seasoned practitioners."

—**GREG JOHNSON, macrobiotic teacher**
and director of the Concord Institute, London

"In *Macrobiotics for Life* Simon Brown presents macrobiotics from his own perspective as well as the different viewpoints of the major world teachers and what the practice means to them. I highly recommend this book to anyone who wants to know more about macrobiotics and anyone who has been practicing it for many years. *Macrobiotics for Life* conveys an open and embracing attitude toward macrobiotics and life in general. Brown is a prolific writer who has once again done an excellent job."

—**FRANCISCO VARATOJO, macrobiotic teacher, author, and consultant,**
and director of the Macrobiotic Institute of Portugal

MACROBIOTICS
FOR LIFE

OTHER BOOKS BY SIMON BROWN

MACROBIOTICS
FOR LIFE

A Practical Guide to Healing for Body, Mind, and Heart

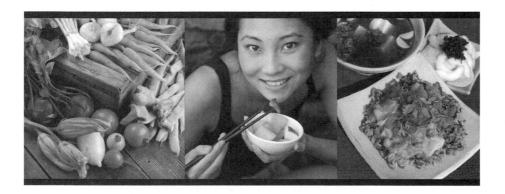

SIMON BROWN

North Atlantic Books
Berkeley, California

Published by
North Atlantic Books
P.O. Box 12327
Berkeley, California 94712

Cover Photos: Left: istockphoto/KCline Photography
Center: istockphoto/Stock Photo NYC
Right: Simon Brown
All interior photos by Simon Brown except "Fresh red, golden, and green vegetables and fruit juices" photo by Dragana Brown
Photo stylists: Melissa Fox and Dragana Brown
Cover and book design by Suzanne Albertson

Printed in the United States of America

Macrobiotics for Life: A Practical Guide to Healing for Body, Mind, and Heart is sponsored by the Society for the Study of Native Arts and Sciences, a nonprofit educational corporation whose goals are to develop an educational and cross-cultural perspective linking various scientific, social, and artistic fields; to nurture a holistic view of arts, sciences, humanities, and healing; and to publish and distribute literature on the relationship of mind, body, and nature.

North Atlantic Books' publications are available through most bookstores. For further information, visit our Web site at www.northatlanticbooks.com or call 800–733–3000.

MEDICAL DISCLAIMER: The following information is intended for general information purposes only. Individuals should always see their health care provider before administering any suggestions made in this book. Any application of the material set forth in the following pages is at the reader's discretion and is his or her sole responsibility.

Library of Congress Cataloging-in-Publication Data

Brown, Simon, 1957–
    Macrobiotics for life : a practical guide to healing for body, mind, and heart / Simon Brown.
        p. cm.
    Summary: "This complete book on the powerful art of macrobiotic healing presents the macrobiotic philosophy, lifestyle choices, delicious recipes, and practical tools for healing the body, mind, and emotions"—Provided by publisher.
    Includes index.
    ISBN 978–1–55643–786–1
    1. Macrobiotic diet. I. Title.
    RM235.B758 2009
    613.2'64—dc22
                                                                2009002427

1 2 3 4 5 6 7 8 9 SHERIDAN 14 13 12 11 10 09

ACKNOWLEDGMENTS

A huge thanks to all those I have worked, played, loved, and hung out with. I feel blessed by being surrounded by people who have been so loving, supportive, generous, stimulating, questioning, challenging, humorous, fun, insightful, colorful, expressive, considerate, and—perhaps most of all—who have been part of that feedback system and told me whatever I needed to hear at the time.

I feel a great affection, gratitude, and respect for everyone in my life and I cherish the times we spend together. Since writing *Practical Wabi Sabi* I have placed a greater value on my interactions with people and felt my own love, affection, and warmth color my exchanges with other humans more deeply than I can remember.

It has been these interactions that have helped shape me and create this book.

CONTENTS

INTRODUCTION

I have written this book as a follow-up to one of my previous books, *Modern-Day Macrobiotics.* While *Modern-Day Macrobiotics* focused on food, this book, *Macrobiotics for Life,* explores the philosophy, thinking, and practices that make macrobiotics such a powerful approach to life.

I have made a point of writing about all the aspects of macrobiotics that are easy to bring into your daily life; these practices of macrobiotics have changed my life and the lives of people I have worked with. I hope you will enjoy a similar transformation.

The foods and recipes in this book use commonly available ingredients and have been specifically designed to be easy to prepare. I have used a language that is clear and understandable, with easy-to-follow suggestions.

Macrobiotics for Life describes a holistic approach to health that shows you ways to explore your body, mind, and heart. You will find practical suggestions on food, meditation, breathing, exercise, thinking, healing, eating habits, your environment, taking responsibility, creating healthy relationships, self-diagnosis, and cooking.

If you want to improve your health and make the most of the rest of your life, trying out the recommendations in this book can help you do it.

PART ONE
THE BEGINNING

If you want to try macrobiotics, it's helpful to understand what you're doing rather than following in blind faith. In this part of the book I will explain what macrobiotics is and how it works. I'll introduce some of the most important macrobiotic ideas for healing. We will explore the way in which holistic healing works, and how healing is ultimately an ongoing process that takes us into all areas of our lives. We'll start a conversation on using our intuition and learning to access our souls. I will talk about self-love and its role in healing, and explain how healing requires a readiness for change and a willingness to be open-minded enough to try out different ways of eating and living. Finally, I will explain how you can get the most out of this book—and therefore out of your adventure into the world of macrobiotics and healing.

CHAPTER ONE

The Essence of Macrobiotic Healing

Macrobiotics amounts to finding our physiological limitations and trying to live within them. This is the cultivation of humbleness. When we think that we can do anything we want, we become arrogant. This arrogance causes sickness.

When we are living within our physical limitations, then our spirituality is free. Macrobiotics seeks freedom in spirit. Freedom exists in our spirits—so we can think anything, but biologically, physiologically we are un-free. We can wish to eat anything we want. But we cannot do it.

Disciplining physical un-freedom is the foundation of spiritual freedom. God didn't give us unlimited biological freedom, but appreciating and taking into consideration our un-free physical condition leads us to greater freedom, both physically and spiritually.

—HERMAN AIHARA, macrobiotic teacher, author, and counselor

HEALING

The dictionary definition of "healing" is: curative, therapeutic, medicinal, remedial, corrective, reparative; tonic, restorative, health-giving, healthful, beneficial. The origin of the words "to heal" is "to make whole."

My definition, and the context of the word as used in this book, is that healing is a process of discovery that brings about change to our selves. Ideally this change will ultimately be one that feels appropriate on all levels. In this sense, it is a continuous journey that takes us through many stages of healing—whether to bring relief from a physical symptom, recover from an illness, sleep better, have more energy, improve digestion, find greater emotional harmony, discover greater meaning to life, or become better connected to our hearts and souls.

Sometimes we may be focused on one pressing health issue, and at other times we might be exploring healing in the biggest sense of the word by looking at what we want to do with the time we have left in our bodies.

Healing the Body, Mind, and Heart

My intention with this book is to provide you with a holistic view of macrobiotic healing that is as complete as possible. I will explain the macrobiotic approach to healing, help you understand how it works, and give you the tools to apply it to yourself.

We will explore healing in terms of the body, mind, and heart. We will consider our physical, emotional, and mental well-being; we will also go further and explore a deeper level, with the soul and spirit.

Macrobiotic healing has evolved over its long history into a holistic approach to health. This is essential, as real healing cannot easily happen by working on one part of the whole. For example, it is difficult to resolve a physical health problem that is caused by stress if we do not take care of the source of the stress itself. We may find foods that can provide temporary relief, but if we do not resolve the cause, the symptoms will inevitably return, even if in a different form.

In *Macrobiotics for Life* we will examine all parts of the whole and look at ways we can engage in our own healing for each.

The Ultimate Healing

Ultimate macrobiotic healing takes us on a continuous journey of self-development that carries us through for the rest of our lives. The big aim is not simply to have more energy or get rid of headaches but to explore the boundaries of what life can be for each of us. There is no long-term point in being healthy for the sake of it. In my macrobiotic view of living a big life, the idea is to have a big dream for what we want to do with our lives, and then use our health to take on that challenge. That is not to say that it cannot happen the other way round: sometimes, through trying to solve a specific health problem we end up on a journey that leads us to a much bigger healing.

In this interpretation, the ultimate healing could be finding that dream, finding something that generates the enthusiasm, desire, hunger for life, and passion that gives you a reason to be healthy and engage in macrobiotics for life. The dream does not have to be anything extraordinary. It could be to be a parent, to write, to play a musical instrument, or to take on community work.

Don't worry if this sounds overwhelming; there is also plenty of help in this book for simply working on something like a headache. My approach is very simple, practical, and easy to follow. It really is a case of one step at a time—and if you're reading this book, you have already taken the first step.

Holistic Healing

If we choose to work with ourselves holistically, then it's important to consider the whole at every stage—to consider what changes we can make in all areas of life to bring about the holistic changes we're looking for. The beauty of macrobiotics is that it is naturally holistic; it is not only steeped in a tradition of holism, but it's constantly evolving and being updated with new ideas to become even more holistic.

We could take different aspects of healing—for example, physical, emotional, mental, social, spiritual, or a connection to the soul—and focus on any one of these at any one time, but if we cannot at some stage work through or embrace them all, our efforts risk being undermined by the parts we left out. In one sense, simply being holistic can be as life-changing as the healing itself.

INTUITION

One of the ultimate aims of macrobiotic healing is to develop our intuition. Intuition is defined as our ability to know something immediately, without the need for conscious reasoning. It is as though our souls, subconsciouses, or inner beings can somehow tap into resources that can guide us through life.

One macrobiotic theory is that our intuition comes from tapping into the forces of nature in a way that brings a certain truth and clarity to a situation. This allows us to step out of our normal logic, learned responses, and reasoning that can confuse us, mislead us, and keep us locked in established patterns of unhelpful behavior or thinking.

One of the ways we suppress our intuition is through beliefs in concepts, dogmas, or rules. If our beliefs are strong enough, we will over rule our intuitive, gut feelings. One of the challenges of writing a book that embraces intuition is that I might unintentionally feed you ideas that, if you believe them enough, will actually make it harder for you to be intuitive and listen to your heart. So, in that spirit, I suggest you bring your intuition up to the surface and see all the ideas here as stepping stones to discovering your own truth. One of my colleagues, Frans Cooper, has a wonderful analogy. When we learn to swim we can start with a life vest or water wings. This helps us get used to the water, work on our swimming techniques, build up confidence, and practice. At some point we can safely discard the vest and swim on our own. If we don't take this step, the vest actually holds us back. It's only when we leave it behind that we can swim fast, dive, and swim underwater.

All the macrobiotic concepts, philosophy, and ideas are similar to a life vest and water wings. They can be very useful and helpful at the beginning to get you up and running with your healing journey, but at some point they will hold you back in terms of developing your intuition and finding the truth of your own healing. For this reason, I would suggest you immerse yourself in this book, learn from the ideas expressed here, try them out, play with them, and begin your experience with macrobiotic healing—but remember, these are all simply a temporary support to get you started.

I do not consider anything in this book to be a universal truth. The ideas here may feel like my truth, but it would be a huge assumption to claim that they will all also be true for you. Each of us is unique, and, ultimately, what works for me will not necessarily work for you. At some stage you will want to free yourself from any conceptual constraints and make macrobiotics yours. I hope you will keep reviewing it and keep finding new ways to make it work for you.

THE JIGSAW PUZZLE

Even though the macrobiotic approach is the most holistic I know of, I am also aware that it is not everything; it's not the whole, assembled jigsaw puzzle of life, but only one piece. I encourage you to explore anything that you think will help you on your journey of self-discovery, in finding your truth about who you are, and in learning what you need to do to live your dream.

CHAPTER TWO

Key Ingredients for Healing

My love of nature and my interest in the philosophy of the Far East came together when I first encountered the writings of George Ohsawa. After I pondered the *Tao Te Ching* through my teens and became enchanted by the Buddhist-influenced beat poets of the 1950s, Ohsawa and Michio Kushi offered practical solutions to my troubled body and soul that changed my life in simple yet profound ways. The patterns of nature that had always seemed external were brought home and connected with my biology as well as my mind and spirit. It is a pity that we are not issued an owners' manual at birth so that we can modify and repair the wear and tear of living; macrobiotics comes close to filling that need when used with a beginner's mind and a sense of humor.

—BILL TARA, macrobiotic teacher, author of *Natural Body Natural Mind*, and head of natural therapies at the SHA Wellness Clinic, Alicante, Spain

In my experience of self-healing and working with people walking through their healing process, there are certain attributes that make the process easier. These can be described most simply as self-love, appreciation, a willingness to change, an open mind, a desire to enter a process of transformation, and commitment.

SELF-LOVE AND APPRECIATION

The healing process starts with self-love. This is so important that Chapter Eighteen is dedicated to developing self-love. It is self-love that gives us the motivation and ability to heal. As esoteric healer Serge Benhayon points out, our souls know only love. It is by connecting with our souls that we find the self-love that too often eludes us.

In macrobiotic books and lectures, the word "appreciation" could be used in this context, but for me self-love is a more current expression that is easier to understand and also easier to feel. This is not the kind of self-love that is about thinking that we are good-looking, clever, wealthy, or cool. It is purely a feeling that we experience when we can connect with the love in our hearts. For that reason we do not need anything more than a connection with our souls to feel it. In fact, for me, any thoughts about who I am and why I would love myself get in the way of connecting with the soul; they stop me from experiencing self-love.

It is particularly helpful to feel self-love regularly when you are working with health issues. It can be easy to drift into feelings of self-loathing, which can contribute to ill health and make it harder to experience our own healing. I would go as far as to say that whatever we do out of the pure feeling of self-love will lead us to a process of self-healing and move us forward in life. For example, if through a moment of stillness and self-love I felt that spending more time with close friends would be healing, then I would follow that impulse, even if it didn't make sense on any other level.

Furthermore, when we feel self-love, we express love. As other people feel our love, we can heal our relationships, friendships and social lives. Self-love can cultivate a gentleness that helps us interact with the world differently and often more kindly. Out of a feeling of self-love we can treat ourselves better and escape our own standards, self-criticism, sense of failure, and unreasonable expectations.

READINESS TO CHANGE

Next most important is a willingness to change. Much of our lives have been spent learning and finding successful strategies. It is a natural human tendency to seek out a successful strategy and then, once found, stick to it. It may even be that your whole personality is made up of the successful strategies you've found at different times in your life. If tantrums get your mother's attention, that becomes a successful strategy; if being the class clown wins you friends, that is another one; if being shy helps you avoid difficult social situations, that is yet another; if being a bully gets you want you want or if taking on a victim mentality wins you sympathy, those are others.

If you can step outside of yourself for a moment and take an honest and critical look inward, you will probably recognize many character traits that you developed at different times in your life to help you succeed. These could include keeping busy, feeling depressed, creating drama, flirting, trying to appear clever, acquiring a wealth of knowledge, being right, and so on. Even alcohol, cigarettes, and other drugs may have initially been a part of someone's successful strategy for making friends, starting relationships, having sex, or creating a special image.

My point here is that many of our successful strategies—which seemed really helpful at one point in our lives—might now be working against us. These learned strategies could be acting as a huge barrier holding us back from making any real change. They could actually be the cause of poor health and unhappiness. Being a clown at school might have worked at school—but it doesn't work in the office. Being self-absorbed and self-obsessed might do something for you as a teenager, but it makes you a pain to be around as an adult. Behavior that got mom and dad rushing to help could have to opposite effect with a husband or wife.

The difficulty we all have is that it's frightening to let go of the very things that have brought us success in the past. And if we did let go of them, who would we be? What would be left? This is why self-love and trusting ourselves is so important. By letting go of our old ways and embracing change, we can begin the journey of our own transformations and, out of that, our own healing.

One of the observations I used in my novel *The Healer* is that when we enjoy a period of success, we tend to want to stay there even if the rest of the world has moved on. I had a great time in my late teens with pubs, parties, and motorcycles; for a while afterwards I was stuck in a pub-going life that was no longer working for me. I wanted to cling to the good times of earlier years, not appreciating that I could move on to even better ones. Once I let go and moved on to something else I got stuck there for a while too, again fearing that letting go would entail a loss.

I find that if I can recognize my own learned strategies and see why I developed them, it's much easier to kiss them goodbye. Somehow that "ah ha!"

moment of realizing why I adopted certain behaviors takes the power out of them, and they become easier to drop.

Being provocative, I would say that any thought about yourself that you feel attached to will hold you back at some point. I could even say that some of the thoughts I was attached to regarding macrobiotics eventually held me back, even after an initial period of great success.

OPEN MIND

A common problem we all have is resistance to change, but keeping an open mind is essential to moving forward. As a child, I never wanted to get in the bath—and then when I was in it I wouldn't want to get out. This kind of resistance seems even more bizarre in adult life, when we realize that we can easily go back to the way things were if a change doesn't work out well for us. There is, for example, no great risk in avoiding foods with added sugar for a month. Nothing can go wrong, nothing will be lost, and you can choose to go back to eating as much sugar as you like when the month is up. What you will have gained is the experience of not eating sugar for a while, and then the experience of eating it again. You will know for yourself what it feels like.

I recommend that anyone reading this book does so with an attitude of "I'll try it for myself and see how I feel." All my ideas and suggestions are simply here for you to try on for while: try on a different perception of yourself and your life for a few days; try on a different way of eating for a few months; try on new breathing, meditation, and exercise practices for a few weeks and experience them for yourself.

TRANSLATION OR TRANSFORMATION

Author Ken Wilber used the phrase "translation or transformation" to differentiate between going through a series of different practices and engaging in ongoing transformation. For example, it would be possible to go from yoga to tai chi to meditation, but take the same set of attitudes from one to the next. We might learn new skills, insights, and techniques each time we take on a new pursuit—but we could translate the same basic patterns of thinking and behavior.

In my work with Serge Benhayon and macrobiotic teacher Greg Johnson, it became apparent that many of the things we turn to, including macrobiotics, can become a mask for avoiding the underlying issues and taking on the process of deep transformation. In a way, it can simply be like finding a new game to play: it might have different rules to learn, but it is essentially another game and therefore part of a process of translation. The challenge for all of us is to put the games to one side, find our own truths, and engage in transformation.

I would encourage anyone embarking on the macrobiotic journey to be open to searching deep inside for the opportunity to transform and keep on transforming. For example, if you find you have a great attraction to coffee, rather than worry about the potential pro and cons of drinking it, use your desire as an opportunity to learn more about yourself and find out why you might be attracted to something that could potentially be harmful. Is coffee taking you away from a state where you could work on yourself? Is it a form of escapism, a distraction from asking questions of yourself?

COMMITMENT FOR LIFE

I liked my publisher's suggestion of calling this book *Macrobiotics for Life* because macrobiotics *is* for life. Not that it needs to be an all-or-nothing diet, or that you will have to spend the rest of your life eating certain foods. Far from it. Macrobiotics is extremely flexible, and I hope you play with until it suits you, and you have the freedom to keep making changes to match your needs in life as they unfold and evolve.

By "for life," I mean that any positive change is about making an investment in yourself for life. This means putting time and, if appropriate, money into transforming yourself. For me this has been through reading books, taking courses, and being around people I feel I can learn from.

Whether you want to call it macrobiotics or not, I feel that if you want to live the biggest life you can, you will benefit from other people's help. And any investment in ourselves is worth infinitely more than any material wealth.

CHAPTER THREE
Understanding Macrobiotics

Each human being is a magnificent breathing masterpiece of life. At birth we have everything we need already: lungs, kidneys, nervous system, liver, skin, etc. Each one of us has an original heart that longs to expand and express itself in a multitude of ways. There is much talk of organic food, organic agriculture, organic housing, etc., but I believe the deeper journey macrobiotics encourages is the restoration of the True Organic Me. It is usually hidden beneath the modern, cultivated, Artificial Me that we acquire over years of mechanical education, dogmatic upbringing, suppressive cultural and familial environments, and profit-driven indoctrination. Practicing macrobiotics doesn't make one better. Each human being is already a living treasure. Macrobiotics offers "art restoration tools" that we can use to restore ourselves when the years of modern cultivation have muted the vibrant colors and brilliance of our human magnificence. We bring forward again the beauty of who we are already: our organic humanness physically, emotionally, mentally, and spiritually. Then, what we can do with our lives, individually and collectively, is beyond measure.

—DAVID BRISCOE, macrobiotic teacher, counselor, and author

After nearly thirty years of working with macrobiotic teachers, counselors, cooks, authors, students, and practitioners, I have attempted to describe what macrobiotics is in terms of the reality of how people practice it rather than a conceptual or idealized model.

DEFINITIONS

Macrobiotics has been an inspiration to so many, people for such a long time, in so many parts of the world, that it inevitably means many different things to different people. To some, it is a healthy way of losing weight and looking good; to others, it is part of a program of recovery from a serious illness. Some people love the philosophy and the way macrobiotics helps connect them to nature. Others revel in its deep spiritual side. And for still others, the foods just taste good—and that's enough. For many it may be part of their desire to improve the ecology of our planet by eating locally grown foods and fewer animal products. (And for someone concerned about animal welfare, a vegan version of macrobiotics is the answer.) Healers say they find that the foods help people feel energy and focus it more easily. Some see macrobiotics as an insurance policy against degenerative disease later in life.

In whatever form macrobiotics is practiced, it embraces the influence food can have on our physical, mental, and emotional health. There is also a wide range of opinions on what eating macrobiotically really entails. One person using macrobiotics to help heal him- or herself from a serious illness might see it as a clean, purist diet of vegetables, grains, beans, seeds, and seasonings; he or she would likely eat from simple lists of the most healing ingredients. Another person might use it to detox, eating miso soup, tofu, steamed vegetables, and brown rice, like a Zen monk; someone else might simply use the principle of yin and yang to define his or her diet and eat much a broader, varied range of natural ingredients while trying to maintain some balance. There are also people who eat macrobiotically by using their intuition for guidance; these people will often have found a core, prime diet that works for them most of the time, but they feel free to eat anything else when they feel it's appropriate.

Furthermore, macrobiotic eating can easily take on the hue of traditional Japanese, Mediterranean, Middle Eastern, or Asian eating styles. In fact, the macrobiotic principles can be applied to the cuisine of any culture. I would claim that macrobiotics is made up of the foods eaten by the healthiest societies from around the world. Macrobiotics is so flexible that vegans and vegetarians, as well as people who enjoy food combining, can adopt it. It can easily be adapted for anyone with a food allergy or digestive disorder.

My interpretation is that macrobiotics is the study of the relationship between humans and their environment. There is an emphasis on food, because, along with air and water, food is where we interact strongly with nature. For many in the macrobiotics movement, how we interact with the energy of our universe is of great importance. This means exploring the effect that lunar phases, seasons, weather, home, clothing, other people, landscapes, food, exercise, and breathing have on our energetic bodies and emotions.

A DIET, A SET OF PRINCIPLES, OR AN UNDERSTANDING?

One of the big discussions within the macrobiotics movement has been whether macrobiotics is a diet, a set of principles for choosing foods, or simply an understanding of food.

I think macrobiotics can be all three. It can start out as a diet, become a way of eating using principles such as yin and yang or the five elements, and eventually turn into an understanding of food where the practitioner has more room to use his or her intuition. Sometimes I might want to go back to it being a diet for a while, and at other times use the principles for a few days—but mostly I enjoy using my intuition to choose my foods.

In *Macrobiotics for Life* I take you through all these possibilities. There are menu plans and recipes in Part Seven and Part Eight, and an explanation of yin and yang along with the five elements in Part Five; by reading the whole book, you will begin to get an understanding of macrobiotics as a whole.

Eating for a Reason

Macrobiotics can be defined as eating for a reason. That reason could be for better health, deep healing, feeding the soul, greater emotional stability, mental clarity, beautiful skin, and so on. Macrobiotic teacher, counselor, and author Michio Kushi would describe it as eating to fulfill our life dreams, to help us do the most we can with the rest of our lives. Which foods might generally suit each of these reasons for eating macrobiotically will be slightly different, and several people eating for a similar reason will all have different individual needs.

Therefore, even if we think of macrobiotics as a diet, it's not a diet that is simple to define. Vegetarianism and veganism have clear, indisputable rules that are easy to follow. Macrobiotics is more flexible—but in this it can be confusing.

The Diet

What all macrobiotics enthusiasts agree on is that at the heart of the macrobiotic diet are whole, unprocessed, living foods, straight from the land. These include a great variety of vegetables; whole grains such as brown rice, barley, quinoa, whole oats, rye, whole wheat, spelt, and corn on the cob; dried beans, including lentils, chickpeas and adzuki beans; fruits, seeds, and nuts; and naturally fermented foods such as miso, shoyu, sauerkraut, pickles, and vinegars. In addition, most people eating macrobiotically will include sea vegetables, oils, tofu, hummus, olives, herbs, mild spices, seasonings, and foods made from processed grains, such as breads, pasta, noodles, couscous, polenta, and muesli. Many macrobiotic people will eat fish and, less often, some eggs, dairy foods, and, occasionally, meat.

In this form, macrobiotics passes all the modern tests for healthy eating. With sufficient vegetables it can easily be slightly alkaline-forming, low in sodium, low in saturated fats, high in monounsaturated oils, low in terms of glycemic index and load, full of nutrients, and vital with living energy.

There is also a strong movement of macrobiotic people who are vegan, eating no animal products at all. Macrobiotics is particularly attractive for people following vegan and vegetarian diets, as fermented soy products (miso, shoyu, tofu, tempeh, and natto) are common in macrobiotic eating and naturally high in iron, calcium, and protein. In its vegan version, macrobiotics is nutritionally complete, except for vitamins B12 and D, for most people, although some can find it harder to absorb iron from purely plant sources.

WHAT CAN MACROBIOTICS DO FOR YOU?

Eating macrobiotically can change your blood chemistry, help you become more alkaline, give you more stable blood sugar levels, build up your mineral reserves, have a healthier intestinal environment, enjoy better digestion, and benefit from regular bowel movements. An alkaline-forming diet can contribute to creating a more alkaline pH in some of our body fluids. This can counter the harmful effects of stress, reduce aches and pains, and improve the function of our immune systems.

In theory, all this can also lead to many other kinds of benefits. During the 1980s and 1990s macrobiotics became known as "the cancer cure diet" due to the many people who wrote about their experiences with macrobiotics and recovery from cancer. People have also used it to manage diabetes, improve arthritic conditions, resolve skin complaints, find greater emotional stability, and help with many forms of degenerative disease.

At the same time, eating macrobiotic foods alone is certainly no guarantee of good health. As I have mentioned, if we don't look at the source of a problem, then food may be only a temporary solution.

CHAPTER FOUR

How Macrobiotics Works

Perhaps the most common reason people begin to eat macrobiotically is because of a fear of sickness and a desire for better health. Unfortunately, it is very difficult to exercise good judgment when such mental pressures drive us. Our thinking and feelings are cramped and strained, because we have not yet been released from our old ways of thinking.

In this first level of macrobiotic eating, most people learn to judge by theory. At this stage, discussions of yin and yang or nutrition are frequent, along with a general tendency towards rigidity.

After a period of strict eating in the beginning, most people find themselves going on a binge, and over-rigidity gives birth to excessive cravings, because of a lack of understanding.

After a while people relax and graduate to the next level. Here they eat by principle. Instead of analyzing every mouthful, they learn to see with a larger viewpoint and enjoy their food more.

Then, if the process continues, we finally achieve the highest level: the recovery of our natural intuition. Up to here we have to study, learn, and make mistakes to acquire insights. At this level, fear has disappeared completely. One is free to eat in a natural human way. Fortunately, the more we eat well the stronger our intuition becomes.

—MICHIO KUSHI, macrobiotic author, teacher, counselor, and thinker for one peaceful world

The dietary aspect of macrobiotics works on different levels. Macrobiotics explores the physical and biological effects of food, air, and water on our bodies, as well as the nutritional and energetic influence food has on our emotions and our thoughts. The idea that foods—particularly whole, living foods—have a living energy of their own, and that this energy can influence the energy inside our bodies to produce different thoughts and emotions is central to macrobiotics. It also has a holistic component that looks at all the possible influences on human health, and tries to bring these into broad alignment in order to bring about a particular change.

BIOLOGY

To explore the biological influence of food, we can follow the path of food through our bodies.

Digestion starts in the mouth. Here the food is physically broken down by our teeth and mixed with our saliva to break down complex carbohydrates. The food we eat will influence the pH reading of our saliva. This in turn will effect our gums and teeth. Essentially, to maintain an alkaline condition in our mouths, about half our daily food intake should be vegetables and some fruit.

Our food is further broken down in our stomachs. Here, an issue is that alcohol and simple sugars are absorbed through the stomach lining straight into the blood, potentially inflaming the lining. In addition, alcohol, foods high in refined sugars, coffee, and some meats can increase acidity in the stomach.

The duodenum is situated below the stomach and at the beginning of the small intestine. Here the food mixes with pancreatic juices and bile from the liver, which has been stored in the gallbladder. The type of food you eat will determine how much of these digestive juices are required. For example, a high-fat diet will place greater demands for bile on the liver and gallbladder.

The small intestine, situated around the navel in the center of your abdomen, is where your food is further broken down and absorbed. The food is absorbed into the bloodstream and taken to the liver for processing. In addition, a gland at the end of the pancreas secretes insulin, which regulates blood sugar, especially to bring down an excess rise due to eating food with a high glycemic index or load. It is also thought that the bones can provide extra minerals to keep the blood from becoming too acidic through stress and overconsumption of acid-forming foods. The blood takes the nutrients to every cell in the body.

There are several organs that take waste from the blood and keep the blood in its optimum condition. The kidneys take out waste, remove excess liquid, and help maintain a blood pH of 7.4. Urine is stored in the bladder, behind the pubic bone, before elimination. You can measure the pH of your urine and discover how it varies according to your diet and stress levels. The lungs bring oxygen to the blood and remove waste, and in the process can influence the pH of the blood. The skin helps eliminate water, salts, and oils.

The spleen is where the blood and lymph meet; it has an important role in the function of the immune system. It also reduces redundant red blood cells.

The heart pumps the blood through the body and is affected by excessive levels of cholesterol attaching to the lining of arteries. This is considered to be worsened by overconsumption of foods high in saturated fats, such as eggs, meat, and dairy products. The risk of cholesterol sticking to the artery lining can be alleviated by eating more monounsaturated fats such as those in fish and olive oil. It is thought that a diet high in vitamin C helps the heart repair itself, reducing the need for the body to produce additional cholesterol to make those repairs.

The reproductive organs can also be influenced by food. Sperm count and quality are thought to be partially influenced by diet, and menstrual cycles can cause food cravings and also respond to changes in diet.

Meanwhile, the food that was not absorbed in the small intestine passes through to the colon, where water is taken out and waste stored in the bowel. A diet high in saturated fats will slow this process and increase the risk of toxins building up along the colon wall. A high-fiber diet cleans the colon lining and reduces the risk of constipation.

ENERGY

The idea that foods have a living energy and that this energy can influence our own energetic bodies comes from traditional Eastern cultures. Indian and Chinese practitioners developed systems to describe the human energetic body. In India, it was the seven chakras; in China, it was a network of meridians and acupressure points.

In either interpretation, the main point to consider is that this energy can be influenced by numerous external factors; when our energies change we feel different, and out of that we experience changes to our thoughts and emotions. At the same time, our thoughts can also change our energetic bodies, creating a two-way interaction.

So, on the one hand, we can say that the weather, lunar cycles, seasons, environment, other people, clothing, atmosphere of a building, and our food can all influence our energy and therefore our states of mind and emotions. On the other hand, we can also override this with our own thoughts and conscious actions. For example, breathing gently and just being aware of the feeling of breathing will change our energetic bodies, regardless of the weather or anything else. However, it is challenging to constantly be in a state of mind that affects our energy in the way we want, so it is helpful to also consider what else is going on around you and how this might change your energy.

I believe that out of all the external influences on us, our food is the easiest to change from one day to the next—and, as we bring food deep into our bodies, it is potentially a powerful energy-changing force. It is common sense to say that if we want to feel calm, centered, and focused, alcohol, sugar, strong spices, and coffee will not help. Macrobiotics takes this further and looks at every food to see how it might influence our energy. We will look at this in detail in Chapter Twenty-One.

CHAPTER FIVE
How to Use This Book

Everything that is and can be languaged is dogma. As long as we maintain a belief that our words express reality, then we will always be imprisoned by some type of dogma. Words do not actually describe real things. Instead, they simply act as fictional divisors of our universe. Beyond this, the universe is really just a nameless "oneness," as explained by Lao Tzu when he wrote:

"The Tao that can be told is not the eternal Tao; The name that can be named is not the eternal name."

When you understand this, then you can have fun and freely play with dogma instead being afraid of it. Dogma is only harmful when we ourselves don't recognize it and then believe something to be so real that we must convince others of it—and even punish them if they don't agree. By the very nature of language, and as we express we create dogma all the time. I am doing it even now as I write this and as you read this.

—PHIYA KUSHI, macrobiotic teacher

I'd like you to use this book to get a complete and holistic understanding of macrobiotics. Therefore, it would help to read the book from the beginning through to end of Part Six. If something does not make sense, relax and keep reading; often, something later in the book will make it easier to see how it all works together and thus get a better understanding of each part.

Once you've read the whole book, you might like to refer back to certain parts to gain a deeper understanding. I hope you'll also find the menu plans and recipes in Parts Seven and Eight useful for ongoing reference.

If you read a part of the book that you disagree with or feel uncomfortable with, relax; try initiating every breath, meditate by feeling each breath, and be aware of how an idea or thought feels to you. In this way you can also read with your heart and be aware of what resonates with you on a deeper level.

Please think of this book as a stepping stone to developing your own truth and intuition. I wouldn't want you to lose your own truth or weaken your intuition by adopting any of my theories, and while you might enjoy trying on a different perception of life and healing for a while, I hope you will use this experience to further your own exploration of yourself.

If you read ideas that challenge a belief or conviction of yours—perhaps a belief you already have about macrobiotics—rather than get caught up in whose idea is right or wrong, explore how you would be different if you embraced either thought. For example, if you believe that macrobiotics is a diet and that certain foods are good for everyone and others harmful, consider how this affects your attitude toward food, how it might influence your relationships with those close to you, and, of course, whether this is really true. You could then compare this to thinking of macrobiotics as an understanding of food, and consider what would be different about your relationships to food and other people if you adopted this thinking.

If you want to bring the ideas in this book into your own life, it's important to actually try them out, to use them in real life. At the end of each chapter I make suggestions for doing so. Ultimately, remember that this book presents my opinions, views, thoughts, and ideas. These are not universal truths, and there's plenty of room for you to make your own interpretation, play with the ideas, and make them your own.

PART TWO
HEALING THE MIND

In this section I will take you though the whole range of macrobiotic ideas that come together and help us heal our minds.

Here you will discover an amazing perception of life to try on and see how you feel. You will find ways to free yourself from stress, negative thoughts, and self-limiting thoughts. You can learn how to live your life as it happens and make the most of every moment. You can, in effect, step out of patterns of thinking that no longer work for you—and into the real you.

I'll describe ways to use your mind to help you heal on all levels, and give you practical ideas on what foods can best feed your mind. In a sense, after reading this section your life will never be the same again, as you will have the choice to see through the self-delusional thoughts that can hold you in unhappiness and keep you from the truth of what's really healing for you.

CHAPTER SIX
Freeing the Mind

At the age of forty-four I came into menopause and the science of energetic truth.

When it happened, I couldn't choose between a feeling of enlightenment and confusion.

I remember a friend writing that there is no real difference between an ordinary person and enlightened one, only that the ordinary person believes experience is concrete, whereas an enlightened person is aware that life is both empty and concrete.

I try to distinguish clearly between myself as the thinker and the vehicle through which I think—the former being consistent in time and space, and the latter being ephemeral. I came to realize that I had spent forty-four years in this life meeting life from reaction, which is a contraction from the fullness of what I am and what I can be.

Living like this had disabled me to stay in my own connection to my inner heart.

I realized that lot of these reactions are unconscious, and before I have even walked out of the house, I can be disconnected from myself by reacting to what someone did or said. I also realized that as a child I was, like the rest of us, burdened with preconceived ideas about things, from my parents, teachers, and others around me.

I became, just like everyone else I knew, programmed to live life by selling my truth for the sake of fitting in with the world and feeling a part of it.

I was in life but not of it.

My biggest challenge remains to resist being pulled into the complex world we live in, which requires an unyielding love and commitment to myself, as well as developing a sense of what is true from within, so that I see the strength of the outer experience for what it truly is.

To detach from the world in order to stay in love is a choice I now make
every moment of every day, with my conscious presence.

—DRAGANA BROWN, co-owner of Luscious Organic

Life can teach us to think in certain ways, and adopt beliefs that prevent us
from thinking freely and being open to change. Sometimes we might hold onto
beliefs that are harmful. If I believe that I need meat for protein, then I won't
do the research to see if it's true; the belief will prevent me from experimenting by not having meat for a few months. Too many rigid beliefs can ultimately
keep us on a very narrow path, where our options to explore, discover, and
experiment are severely limited. Part of the process of healing our minds is
seeing if we can let go of some of our beliefs and gently bring greater mental
freedom into our lives.

NON-CREDO

George Ohsawa embedded the idea of non-credo into macrobiotic philosophy. Non-belief is a core element of Indian Buddhist, Chinese Taoist, and
Japanese Zen Buddhist philosophy. "Credo" comes from the Latin for "I
believe"; Ohsawa talked about non-credo in terms of developing an endless
curiosity. You may remember that when you were a child, you had questions
about everything; Ohsawa encourages us to rekindle that attitude. The idea is
not to find answers, but to be engrossed in the process of discovery, exploration, and inquiry. Ultimately, the solution is to find out more about ourselves
and our relationships with the world around us rather than having a list of
beliefs or universal truths.

For me, the idea of non-credo applies to man-made ideas, concepts, dogma,
principles, theories, and doctrines rather than belief in oneself, feelings, intuition, or any kind of connection to the soul.

How Does This Affect Our Practice of Macrobiotics?

A non-credo approach to life is the essential counterbalance that can reduce
the risk of becoming dogmatic, overly reliant on theories, and even fanatical

with our practice of macrobiotics. Non-credo can help us be imaginative, creative, and intuitive with our cooking. Perhaps most important, non-credo encourages us to practice macrobiotics from our own hearts, and not someone else's belief system; for me, this is the nugget of gold in George Ohsawa's philosophy.

Here are some questions to consider and to help you see how you might be influenced by your beliefs, if you still have any!

Does One Belief Exclude Other Thinking?

Once we take on a belief, is there a risk that we'll find it harder accept a contrary belief at the same time? Can the human mind believe in two opposing truths simultaneously? If not, it would seem that the more beliefs we have, the smaller our world becomes, as each new belief means we will exclude millions of other possible thoughts—making us micro- rather than macrobiotic. Does having lots of beliefs make us narrow-minded, defensive, tribal, and self-righteous as we hang onto what's in our minds and try to align with similar people?

Do Beliefs Get in the Way of Intuition?

If we believe in too many concepts, do we overrule our intuitive feelings if they don't match our treasured beliefs? For example, if we have memories of all the foods we've ever eaten and a deep biological knowledge of how these foods affect us, what happens when our bodies cry out for a certain food to address a nutritional deficiency, but it's not part of our version of the macrobiotic diet? Rather than develop our intuition and creativity in general, do beliefs stunt this powerful side of our beings?

Can Beliefs Make Our Minds Smaller?

If we were walking along a busy shopping street and a pink elephant flew by, we would see it—but most of us would not register it in our minds, because a flying pink elephant is not within our belief systems. If we had a young child with us, he or she would look at it excitedly, because, for a young mind, flying pink elephants are possible. This invites questions: As we take on more beliefs, are we imprisoning are minds in narrow channels of thinking? Do we lose out on all the amazing, wonderful, beautiful, mind-blowing things that are going on outside of our belief systems? Are we limited by our beliefs?

Is It Possible That Beliefs Stunt Our Development?

When we take on a belief, do we then stop any inquiry, search, or discovery, and halt our own development? If, for example, I believed that eating macrobiotic foods would solve all my problems, and I ate only macrobiotic food, would I still make the effort to form better relationships, be physically fit, and learn from other people? When we take on a belief, do we tend to see the subject as closed instead of continuing to explore it?

Do We Need to Believe in Something to Do It?

Will someone take on the effort to eat macrobiotically if he or she does not believe in it? If macrobiotics is a creative, artistic, intuitive way of exploring the relationship between food, emotions, and health then is it possible that beliefs might just get in the way of that journey? If macrobiotics is a science, with the aim of developing the ultimate healthy diet, then beliefs may be required if your expectation is a long life and freedom from illness. But is macrobiotics a science, and is the idea that you can prevent or cure illness through macrobiotics totally true? Do we need to believe in music, art, film, fiction, food, friendships, sex, and love in order to enjoy them and feel improved by experiencing them?

Why Have Beliefs?

There must be a reason we like to find things to believe in—otherwise, why we would we have that desire in our characters? The most common and researched advantage of having a belief is the placebo effect. If a group of people believe that miso soup will help them recover from pain, about a third of the people in the group who eat miso soup will typically show signs of improvement from that belief alone. The belief might be strengthened by some kind of theory, whether yin and yang or something more scientific. Someone else having exceptionally good results eating miso soup will further strengthen the belief that miso soup will be the answer. It then becomes a point of discussion as to whether we need to believe in something outside of ourselves in order to get that placebo effect, or is self-love and belief in ourselves enough?

There is also the nocebo effect to be considered, where believing that a certain food is bad for us. Such a belief increases the risk of suffering as a result of eating a so-called "bad" food. For example, if I believe that eating sugar makes me hyperactive, then that belief increases the risk that I will feel hyperactive after eating sugar.

I think we've all experienced difficult times and found that beliefs get help get us through them—but do the same beliefs then work against us if we then cling to those ideas after they have served their purpose?

PRACTICAL EXERCISES

1. Write a list of ten things you believe in. Next to each belief, write down how it might affect you. Include aspects you enjoy and those you might want to be free from.

   For example:

   I believe I am what I eat.

   Feels good knowing I am becoming healthy through eating natural, organic foods. Helps me avoid less healthy foods.

   Might lead to being obsessive about food and limit my social life.

   Could introduce negative thoughts about myself if I eat something processed and sugary.

   Use this simply to create an awareness of the beliefs you have and that there will be benefits and disadvantages in healing them.

2. Choose a subject that interests you. See how far you can take your interest on the basis of asking questions. See where asking why, how, when, and where takes you. Remember to resist looking for answers; instead, seek to develop you power of inquiry. Try to enjoy the process of exploring a subject.

3. Try releasing yourself from a chosen belief. For example, if I believed I had to wash organic vegetables before eating them, I could experiment by living without that belief, washing my vegetables if I felt like it and

not if I didn't. Then, after a few weeks of being free from that belief, see if you have a more intuitive response to the issue. In my example, I might find I begin to feel that unwashed organic vegetables actually are better for me.

4. Make a list of things you do not do because of your beliefs. For example, if I believe that letting my children watch television is bad for them, it would stop me from cuddling up on the sofa with them and watching a comedy.

5. See if you have a belief that is affecting your health and make a note of it. For example, if I believed that I had to look a certain way and this caused me a lot of stress, my belief could be harming me. Play with the idea of dropping that belief. In my example, I might imagine myself going out dressed in whatever I felt like wearing and feeling good about myself regardless of what other people think.

SUMMARY

1. George Ohsawa introduced the principle of non-credo, or non-belief, to macrobiotic philosophy.

2. Non-belief is a core element of Indian Buddhist, Chinese Taoist, and Japanese Zen Buddhist philosophy.

3. By adopting beliefs, we close our minds to other possibilities and make our world smaller.

4. The more beliefs we have, the harder it becomes to use our intuition and find our own truths.

5. Living out someone else's beliefs prevents us from being ourselves and living our own truths.

6. Rigid beliefs can stop our own evolution and growth.

7. Negative beliefs may harm us.

8. Some beliefs can lead to stress and negative emotions that prevent us from healing.

9. Beliefs can be motivating.

10. Beliefs can help us through hard times.

CHAPTER SEVEN
Assumptions, Expectations, and Relationships

I feel quite uncomfortable with the word "healer"—at least for myself. It suggests that I am doing something to someone when, in my work, it's about making space for the other person to really, really be. I'm not that good at shifting energy, but when I remember that I am nothing—that I am literally more space than matter—and I relax into that truth, energy just shifts, in me, and in the person I'm working with. Whether it's taking someone into hypnosis, or teaching a macrobiotic class, I just ask the universe to flush my psychic toilet and release all the ego poo-poo floating about. What a relief to surrender to the great nothingness, which is the great everythingness! So empty, and yet so full. That is where, I believe, healing occurs.

—JESSICA PORTER, macrobiotic teacher and cook, and author of *The Hip Chick's Guide to Macrobiotics*

One of the challenges of being human is that we tend to muddle up reality with things we make up in our heads. When we start to believe the made-up thought, we risk becoming deluded. In one sense, this is fine—that is, if we are happy with our made-up thoughts. But if those thoughts are making us unhappy, they can make our healing journeys more difficult and even sabotage the good work we put into eating healthy foods, exercising, and meditating.

One definition of mental health could be our ability to tell the difference between reality and self-made thoughts: to be able to recognize opinions, views, ideas, and theories for what they are, and not to think they describe reality. This philosophy is rooted in Taoist and Buddhist thinking. Author Byron Katie presents the ideas in an easy-to-use format in her book *Loving What Is*.

ASSUMPTIONS

I'm often amazed at how easy it is to confuse reality with thoughts we have made up in our heads. This applies to relationships more than anything; it's common for us to make an assumption about someone else and think it's reality. For example, a colleague might criticize me or say something with a certain attitude, and in the past I might have read into it that he disliked me, disapproved of what I was doing, or found me irritating. The situation would have become much worse on the occasions I went on to think my assumption was true. In reality, I did not really know what my colleague thought. Maybe one of my assumptions was true, but it just as likely could have been that he had a headache, had just had a fight with his wife, or was incredibly constipated.

I notice that relationships, families, and close friendships can end up encompassing many assumptions. These are most apparent when they become absolutes. "She always nags me," "He never helps around the house," "She doesn't understand me," "He doesn't care about me anymore." Of course, it's highly unlikely that anything is always or never true in reality.

The big question isn't whether our assumptions are right or wrong, but how they affect us. As we'll see later, there may not be any right or wrong anyway. So if we make an assumption and believe it, and it makes us angry, we need to ask ourselves whether we want that feeling. If not, why make the assumption?

It's possible that if our assumptions cause us to feel angry, jealous, depressed, fearful, anxious, or stressed, those assumptions might be making us ill. It may be that no real healing will take place while we are still living out those assumptions and suffering from those emotions. The sad part of this is that assumptions are self-made; we're doing it to ourselves.

MEANINGS

Not only do we make assumptions, but we also give those assumptions meaning. For example, I might make the assumption that if I'm late for an appointment, the woman I'm meeting will be upset with me. I could then go on to make that mean I am useless, always late, or unreliable. Again, this is completely self-made—I'm doing it to myself. If I use being late as a learning experience and work out how to be on time in the future, there might be some value in it, but to simply feel a sense of failure is potentially unhealthy.

It's common for people in relationships to give meaning to other people's actions: "If he really loved me, he would buy me a new ring"; "If she loved me, she would look after me." Again, these are wild assumptions and not grounded in reality. True love is not conditional, and does not rely on someone doing something to prove it. The meanings you give events are always your choice and your creation. If they hurt you, then try not having them. Try living in the moment and in reality.

EXPECTATIONS

When we expect something to happen and it doesn't, we have an unmet expectation. Unmet expectations can be a great source of disappointment, anger, and frustration. For example, I might expect this book to sell well and then feel disappointed if it doesn't, or I might expect my children to do their homework and feel let down when they forget.

Our use of the words "should" and "shouldn't" are often a sign of an expectation. If a woman says, "He should be more understanding," it shows her expectation of how her boyfriend should behave. Again, it's fine to have expectations if they make you happy, but if those expectations bring unwanted and possibly unhealthy emotions, then you have to ask yourself: Is it worth it? How will these expectations affect my journey and my process of healing?

I have had discussions where people express that there would be no point in living without expectations. To me this indicates they are not happy with themselves as they are. If we live in the moment, connect with our souls, and find self-love, expectations about the future become less of an issue. In fact, thinking about the future and having expectations can take us out of living our lives as they happen. All the time spent creating expectations and worrying about them distracts us from enjoying the moment.

A lot of expectations can be cultural, social, or learned from our parents. A woman may expecting her husband to do certain things because of her experiences growing up with her father. Similarly, a man may create expectations of his lover through seeing how his mother behaved in her relationship with his father. Growing up in England, I might have certain cultural expectations that would not work in the United States.

SHOULD AND SHOULDN'T

Again, two words we use when we make assumptions and that suggest an expectation are "should" and "shouldn't": "You should be more romantic," "You shouldn't go out with your friends," "You should take me out more." There are no universal rules about what someone should or shouldn't do. These words invite argument, as my shoulds and shouldn'ts will be different from yours. We can quickly deteriorate into a discussion on who has the most righteous shoulds and shouldn'ts.

If you catch yourself using these words when talking, you have wandered into the realm of making assumptions and having expectations. More helpful ways to express the same opinions are, "I would like us to be more romantic together," "I feel insecure when you go out with your friends," and "I would like you to take me out more." With this language, you are simply expressing your own feelings rather then making assumptions.

COMPARISONS

It's part of our nature to compare ourselves to others. But, as with assumptions, this also invites unhappiness. If I compared myself to one of my friends and came to the conclusion that he was better looking, wealthier, and more entertaining, where would that leave me? Not in a self-loving space that would help me pursue my journey in life. If I could somehow use the comparison to make changes to my life—for example, if I noticed that my friend ate a healthy diet or had an interesting fitness program—there would be some value in learning from the comparison; otherwise, comparisons become a form of emotional self-abuse.

HABITS

Assumptions, expectations, and comparisons become habits, and after a while, we come to see them as reality. For example, we can end up believing that it is fact that the woman in a relationship should cook the meals. Breaking out of these habits is a challenge. Sometimes habits become so deeply ingrained that we can no longer see any other option. In our minds, what is really an opinion has become something we believe in and, in effect, a universal truth or fact.

BREAKING FREE

The beginning of the process of breaking free of making assumptions and giving things meanings is to recognize what you are doing. The biggest change will come about by simply noticing that you have made an assumption. Once you can separate out what is real, the rest loses its power as you realize that it is just your own thoughts, opinions, and views. It is a choice, and if you don't like the way you feel with a particular thought, you are free to change it.

Once we recognize that we are making assumptions, we can catch ourselves and remind ourselves that they're just opinions. If we start to create an expectation, we can check whether we really want to go down the path that may result in disappointment or frustration.

In my experience, the more I do this the easier it is to stay in the reality of situations. I find relationships so much more fulfilling when I can fully interact with the other person openly and honestly, rather than being distracted from the moment with a head full of assumptions and expectations.

MOVING FROM YOUR HEAD TO YOUR HEART

Assumptions, expectations, and meanings tend to reside in our heads. One way to see them differently is to move out of our heads and focus on our hearts. There is a simple breathing and meditation you can use to help this process.

Start by consciously initiating every in and out breath. Once you have started each breath, let the rest of it follow naturally. There is no need to breath deeply, slowly, or in any special way. When you're comfortable starting every breath, try to feel everything you can about breathing. Feel the air, your chest, and your abdomen move; feel the rhythm of your breathing. As you do this, be aware of your heart and chest and, with that, be aware of how you feel. Recognize the emotions you have.

If you find you start thinking about something, be aware of the thought, and then go back to feeling your breathing.

PRACTICAL EXERCISES

After each exercise, I give examples based on real-life situations that I have experienced.

Assumptions

1. Each time you experience an unwanted emotion, separate reality from whatever you have made up in your head.
2. Write out what happened. Ask yourself whether all of it is completely true, and write out how certain aspects may or may not be true.
3. If you can recognize the parts that are your own assumptions, ask yourself whether you feel happy with them. If not, try *not* making the assumption, and write out how you feel.
4. If you feel that your perspective on what happened is completely true and there is no other possible interpretation, ask yourself what meaning you assigned to it. Write it down. Is this meaning completely true? If the meaning you came up with is creating unwanted emotions, try not believing it, and write out how you feel.
5. Try your breathing meditation to take a rest from everything that's going on in your head, and see if through your heart you feel differently about an issue.

One Example

What happened?

My wife came home and was angry at me for listening to my music too loudly. I felt resentful, as she could have been more loving.

Is this true?

It's possible she had a stressful time at work, and she suffers from headaches—so she might have been angry about the situation she was in rather than angry with me.

How do I feel now?

I feel more sympathetic toward her and I want to help her relax.

Another Example

What happened?

I asked my son to tidy the house while I was out. When I came back, it was still a mess.

Is this true?

Yes, this was true.

What meaning did I assign to it?

I felt he did not care about me and did not appreciate everything I did for him.

Is this meaning true?

No, I do not know this to be true. He is loving and affectionate at other times.

How do I feel?

Better able to remind him to tidy up calmly and with love.

Expectations

1. When feeling any kind of unwanted emotion during or after an interaction with someone, write out what happened.
2. Write out how you felt.
3. Write out what your expectation of the person was.
4. Write out how you would feel if you didn't have the expectation.

An Example

What happened?

I spent all day looking for gift for my wife, and bought her a beautiful black woolen sweater. When I gave it to her, she asked if I would mind if she chose something else, as she is very fussy about what she wears.

How did I feel?

I felt a sense of failure and that I had not made her happy.

What was my expectation?

I expected her to be excited and happy and to love the sweater.

How do I feel without the expectation?

I can respect that she doesn't want to waste money on something she doesn't feel comfortable wearing, and I would enjoy going shopping with her to choose something she would wear more often.

Expectations of Ourselves

1. When feeling any unwanted emotion about yourself write out what happened.
2. Write out how you felt.
3. Write out what your expectation was.
4. Write out how you would feel without the expectation.

What happened?

I went to give a talk, and there were only ten people there.

How did you feel?

I felt unappreciated, and that my work was not getting the recognition it deserved.

What was my expectation?

I expected the room to be full of people wanting to listen to my talk.

How do I feel without the expectation?

Better able to appreciate the people who did come to listen to me. I realized it was arrogant for me to expect anyone to turn up, and that I could have a really meaningful time with the people who were there.

SUMMARY

1. Taoist and Buddhist thinking teaches us to separate reality from self-made thoughts. Mental health can be defined as ability to do this.
2. We talk and think in terms of opinions, views, and thoughts. These are unlikely to be universal truths.
3. Humans tend to make assumptions about each other, and this can distract us from enjoying our interactions.
4. Sometimes our assumptions lead us into experiencing unwanted and potentially unhealthy emotions.
5. We may give events a meaning that is harmful to us.
6. Expectations increase the risk of unwanted emotions.
7. Thinking that someone should or shouldn't do something signals that we have made assumptions and have expectations.
8. Comparisons with other people can be self-destructive and prevent us from enjoying our self-love.
9. Making assumptions and having expectations can become an entrenched habit.
10. The key to breaking free of assumptions and expectations is to recognize when you have them and to see them as opinions, speculation, and views rather then as facts.
11. If your assumptions and expectations contribute to your feeling unhappy, try to let them go.

CHAPTER EIGHT
Responsibility

I was floored when I discovered that I, a macrobiotic counselor, had breast cancer. I was supposed to be immune, yet it was happening to me. I had to employ conventional methods of slashing and poison to open myself up physically until I had time to do so spiritually. Then I began the real healing. I took full responsibility and saw my illness as a way to heal my life. I looked at my relationships, my fear of lack, my shortcomings, and my strengths. I joined groups, conducted workshops, practiced imagery and meditation—in short, I did whatever interested and excited me. It became a wonderful journey and I thank God for this opportunity to grow and develop.

—GINAT RICE, macrobiotic teacher, cook, and counselor,
and author of *Macrobiotic Meals* and *Healing Stories*

George Ohsawa emphasized taking responsibility for everything that happens in our lives. He had little sympathy for people who express a victim mentality. Here, responsibility means taking control of our lives, making decisions without seeking approval, and accepting responsibility for our past actions.

Simply by taking responsibility for our own health, we can experience greater healing. The "I'm going to take control of my own life and health" attitude in itself can be enough to make an improvement to our health, even before we start to take action.

BEING RESPONSIBLE FOR YOUR HEALTH

When George Ohsawa's book *Zen Macrobiotics* was published in English in 1960, the idea of being responsible for our own health was considered irresponsible. At that time, people tended to go about their normal routine and, if ill, to follow the doctor's advice. The current practice taking responsibility for our own health now seems obvious.

The macrobiotic approach to being responsible is to find the kind of foods, exercise, and lifestyle that will keep us in good health; to be able to make adjustments should this not be sufficient; and to adapt to our changing circumstances.

In my experience, this is a lifetime's work. As I grow older, new challenges appear, and I notice that I am continually learning from these experiences—and, as a result, adjusting my way of life. For example, I started eating macrobiotically when I was twenty, partly to overcome gout. This was highly successful, and I had no further experience of gout until much later. As a result of the later attack, I looked into the effects of food on my acid and alkaline balance. Using test strips, I monitored my pH balance and found that the style of macrobiotic eating I was using had become acid-forming. By greatly increasing my vegetable consumption, I was able to become more alkaline. I was then free from further gout for many years. One recent summer, I experienced oversensitivity to the sun and a further gout attack. (It may even be that my sun-sensitivity and gout were linked: Gout is largely caused by an increase in uric acid, which is produced by the body to repair DNA. In my case, the sun could damage my DNA and the gout could be a side effect of my body repairing itself.) These events encouraged me to go to an esoteric healing course with Serge Benhayon, which changed my life and prompted me to explore deeper emotional issues that were influencing my physical health. Now another year has passed without any gout, and if it ever comes back I can keep working on myself.

Another incident from my past was finding, some years ago, that I was beginning to develop hemorrhoids. These are also quite possibly one of the body's amazing mechanisms that help us maintain health—in this case, releasing blood that might otherwise damage the colon. When organic dark chocolate became widely available, I started eating some regularly in the evenings. Friends and family, including my former brother-in-law, Denny Waxman, helped me realize that the chocolate was not helping my health. But found that I could stop for only a week or two; then I would find an excuse to start again. It was after the healing course that my desire melted away; if I'm ever tempted now, simply going into my gentle breathing is enough to defuse the need. As a result, the hemorrhoids receded.

I use these experiences from my own life to illustrate how we can all take responsibility for our health, and through that not only relieve specific symptoms but also greatly enhance our lives in many other ways. With the Internet, research, books, courses, and a general greater awareness of healing it has become much easier to be responsible for our health—which also means seeing a doctor for regular checkups and, if appropriate, getting a professional diagnosis for any ailments.

TAKING CONTROL

George Ohsawa talked about being free to take control of our lives. When I started practicing macrobiotics, it had a pioneering spirit dictating that we should (note the word "should" and the expectation that goes with it!) be able look after ourselves, independent from big business. This is part of what inspired me to start my own engineering design business and, later, help run a macrobiotic center in Philadelphia with Denny Waxman, followed by a much larger center in London. At that time, the macrobiotic community carried out a lot of the natural food processing themselves. People even made their own futons and, of course, grew vegetables.

As a result of all this, I felt a great feeling of being in control of my life. Previously I had worked in large companies where I was told what to do each day and had very little control over my working life. It wasn't until I started practicing macrobiotics that I could take any control over my health. Before it had just seemed like bad luck if I got a headache or indigestion. It was through this feeling of being in control that I realized I had a greater influence over my own destiny than I ever imagined. I sensed the opportunity that I really could make the most of the rest of my life. This brings us back to George Ohsawa's idea that macrobiotics is all about living the biggest life possible, and to do that we need to see how much control we can take over our lives.

This doesn't mean we can't live a full life working for a big corporation, but it does suggest that no matter what situation we find ourselves in, we can explore ways to take greater control.

LIVING OUR OWN LIVES

Being responsible also implies making our own decisions and living our own lives. If you feel unable to do something without other people's approval, then you have given them a degree of control over your life. Living your own life means feeling confident enough to do what genuinely and intuitively feels right. If you have the conviction to do something and you do it out of love for yourself and any others involved, you can find a way to be true to yourself while also being considerate, gentle, and empathetic. In terms of healing, this might involve making a decision to try something that feels right to you even though other people disagree or advise you against it.

Just as we can lose control of our own lives to others, we can also lose our own power by trying to control someone else's life. We can try to run our own lives—and several other people's at the same time. This is common in romantic relationships, and between parents and their children. We might try to make decisions for our loved ones, tell them what to do, or even interfere with their choices. Two things happen: first, you make it harder for the other person to live his or her life; second, you dilute your ability to live your life, as you have to drag everyone else along with you.

When you try to run someone else's life and you want to make a change in your own life, there's a temptation to try and change everyone else at the same time. This has been a recurring theme in macrobiotics; for example, a mother starts eating macrobiotically and puts a huge effort into getting her husband and children to change their diets. This course of action can cause relationship problems, as family members feel under attack and react badly, making it harder to experience healing on all levels—body, mind, and heart.

My view is that it is better to live our own lives. If, in response to our own choices, people close to us want to join in, that's fine; but it's important to also accept that they might not, and feel good about either situation. Being parents of young children is an exception; in that case, we do have a responsibility to look after others, including providing them with a wide variety of natural, healthy foods.

ACCEPTING RESPONSIBILITY

If we're taking control of our lives, it also means taking total responsibility for our actions and not blaming anyone else if something goes wrong. I notice that sometimes it's easier to go along with the crowd, knowing that if there are problems I will not be held responsible. If I'm honest with myself, I must admit that I sometimes don't stand up and lead with power because of this tendency.

Being responsible suggests being able to admit to our mistakes and correct them, being ready to apologize and willing to see how we might have contributed to a difficult situation. By being the first to take responsibility when other people feel upset by our actions, we can reduce the risk of resentment. In the past I have felt I would lose face, show weakness, or be taken advantage of—but I have come to realize through my life partner Dragana's example that being able to apologize is a strength.

ETHICS, MORALS, AND HONESTY

Christoph Wilhelm Hufeland, the founder of macrobiotics (see The History of Macrobiotics in Part Five), considered morals to be an important part of his lifestyle for longevity. Part of the Taoist tradition is based on doing the right thing, living out your own ethics and morals. Buddhist thought includes the idea that whatever we do we leaves imprints on other people, and in order to live ethically we would therefore consider what kind of imprints we do and don't want to leave. I would suggest that creating your own morals and ethics works most easily if it comes out of a state of self-love in which you also feel a natural love for everyone and everything else.

It's not for me to tell you what your ethics should be; I hope you'll complete the exercise below and find your own. However, I can tell you that in all the religions, spiritual movements, and philosophies I am aware of, honesty is a common feature. This takes us back to living in the real world and limiting how deluded we let ourselves become, because honesty starts with ourselves. If we're honest with ourselves, then we have one characteristic in place that can bring about our healing. Without honesty we lose an essential feedback system. If we lie to ourselves about what we have eaten or whether we exercise or not, we're no longer are in touch with the reality of what's happening, and we cannot build up our intuition based on experience. Our learning and self-development become misplaced, built on untruths.

If we live a life of lies, even small lies, it becomes more difficult to build up our wisdom as we get older. Wisdom comes with age because it is built on the sum of all our experiences—but if those experiences aren't true, then what kind of wisdom do we create? A lack of honesty even affected the macrobiotics movement during the 1980s and 1990s. An inability to be honest with ourselves and each other when aspects of the diet were not working, or when unsubstantiated claims were being made, meant that the natural evolution of macrobiotics was slowed, because we pretended everything was fine when—if we were honest—there was plenty of room for improvement.

COLLECTIVE RESPONSIBILITY

The other side of taking responsibility for ourselves is collective responsibility. In one sense, it's easy to take responsibility for our own lives and leave everyone else to live theirs. This becomes complicated when we introduce the idea that we are all connected, and every action we make affects other people. If we embrace this idea, then the effects of our actions on other people become part of our collective responsibility.

This contradicts the idea that we can take total responsibility for our lives, as it suggests that if we are connected and can influence other people, then the reverse must also be true. Part of the challenge here is to be able to accept contradictory ideas at the same time. This may sound like a ridiculous notion, but when it comes to healing there is simply no need for all of our ideas to line up neatly; it's fine to have a collection of ideas that help you live your life even if, for now, it seems illogical. In my experience, we can be in a state where we are closely connected to nature and, once in that centered, soulful state, we're less influenced by other people even though we may be influencing them.

For my own ethics, I chose to treat people with compassion, respect, and dignity in order to try and ensure my own imprints are as I would like them to be. Being gentle with people is another way to ensure that we can live our lives while taking a broader responsibility for our actions.

Collective responsibility enables us to take on much bigger projects than we could manage on our own. Trying to limit global pollution, encourage peace, or increase organic farming is easier when we adopt the concept of collective responsibility.

Responsibility Abuse

The idea of me being responsible for myself can be abused if I then take the attitude that other people are responsible for themselves. I made the choice to live my life the way I have and to take the responsibilities I have. In my choice of ethics, it wouldn't be appropriate to apply my principles to others and say that their problems are their responsibility and therefore not my problem. Responsibility then becomes an excuse not to help out or be compassionate or sympathetic. This kind of attitude disconnects us from other people, which can in itself be unhealthy.

MORNING MEDITATION

In the morning, you can try this meditation to think about the kind of imprints you want to create during the day. Start by consciously initiating every in and out breath while absorbing yourself in feeling every breath. When you feel still, consider how you would want to live this day if it were your last. If this were your last day in this body, what kind of interactions would you want, which aspects of your character would you want to shine through, and what would you choose not to be?

PRACTICAL EXERCISES

1. Write out three areas of your life you can take control over. For example, you might choose some of the following: your food, your exercise routine, what you wear, what you do in the evenings, your meditation practice, whether to smoke or drink alcohol, when you go to sleep, how much television you watch, how much time you spend on the computer, and when you're going to relax and how. Plan out how you will take responsibility for the three areas you choose.

2. Write down anything you want to do but haven't because you're sensitive to someone else's opinions. Write out how you want to communicate your intention to that person so that it is expressed gently and with love, but also comes from a quiet inner confidence.

3. Write down three ways you try to run other people's lives. Think about how you can take responsibility for no longer doing those things.

4. Write out three incidents where you contributed to someone else becoming upset, and think out how you can communicate an apology.

5. Write out a list of ethics for how you want to treat other people. This might include honesty, compassion, integrity, dignity, respect, love, gentleness, kindness or anything else you can think of. Keep this in a highly visible place for a while to remind yourself of your commitment to this way of being with people.

6. Write down any project that you can become involved in where you can participate in taking collective responsibility. This might be helping at the local school, looking after the elderly, joining a green or ecological movement, or getting involved in an aid project.

7. When you wake up, meditate on how you would want to be today if it were your last day.

SUMMARY

1. George Ohsawa recognized that taking responsibility for our own lives is one of the prime steps to better health.

2. Taking responsibility for your health is a lifetime's work of continual self-reflection and adjustment.

3. Taking control of our lives helps us be the master of our own destinies.

4. Have the confidence to live your own life without feeling the need for approval.

5. Avoid running someone else's life.

6. Accept responsibility for your mistakes and be ready to apologize.

7. Write out a list of ethics you want to live by.

8. Consider the kind of imprints you want to leave on other people.

9. Honesty is essential to developing wisdom.

10. Explore taking collective responsibility and joining in with group projects.

11. Be aware that the principle of total responsibility can lead to a form of abuse where, rather than being sympathetic, we think another person's suffering is their problem.

CHAPTER NINE

Letting Go of Limiting Thoughts

On holistic thinking: If you have one of something and split it in two, the one becomes limited in relation to its original state. We could use a lump of clay as an example. If you have a big mass of clay (Tao) and you split it in two (yin and yang), the mind perceives this as a duality, where in actuality it's just one hunk of clay. If you shape the first piece of clay into a figure of an angel and the second into a figure of a devil, the mind will say, "The angel figure is good, and the devil figure is bad." In reality it is neither; it is a lump of clay. The mind's perception of the shape created the problem—not the clay. You are not able to see the clay for what it truly is—hence, being deluded by creating a good and a bad.

—ANDY NICOLA, Asian divination consultant and author of *The Luo Shu Oracle*

It's natural to adopt thoughts that can limit our thinking as we grow up. The problem with having a fixed mind is that our options in life become reduced, and our attachment to thoughts can even prevent us from taking a course of action that would be healing.

Fixed thinking is often centered on thinking in terms of good and bad or right and wrong, and being judgmental. This is not the same as having our own ethics; instead, it's trying to classify things such as food, people, or lifestyles. Fixed thinking can cause us the greatest harm when we develop ideas that we want to become universal truths. Rather than thinking that eating an apple is good for me, it is when I go on to think that eating apples is good for everyone, that it is a universal truth, that I become deluded, lose my honesty, and become disconnected from reality.

MENTAL FLEXIBILITY

Rather than trying to label things as good or bad, I suggest it would be healthier to understand things and see when they might be helpful to you and when they might work against you. This understanding will be personal to each of us, and it will come through a deeper exploration of how we interact with our environments. With this approach, it's harder to generalize for everyone or to think in terms of absolutes.

For example, I might find that eating a miso soup everyday helps me digest my food more easily—but to then expect this to go on forever and/or to expect everyone else to have the same experience would show that I was getting stuck in a fixed mindset.

Good and Bad

Thinking in terms of good and bad is a familiar human trait. We want to learn the rules and find out what's correct and what's not. This is common in macrobiotics; practitioners want to know what the good and bad foods are.

The problem with this thinking is that we're all different, and the foods that work best for me may not be the same as those that work best for you. We may find we have a lot in common and to help get started you might find eating the same kind of foods that I eat will help for a while; but ultimately it would not make sense to limit yourself to my current diet. In addition, over time your needs might change, and if you're stuck with a rigid list of good and bad foods, you won't be able to adapt and continue your process of learning from your real life experience of eating different foods.

Rather than thinking in terms of good and bad, I think in terms of what works best for me in particular situations. In my experience, lots of vegetables, salads, and fruit helps me feel cooler. Soups, stews, and juices can be deeply relaxing. Porridge, noodles, or certain breads can be energizing. So rather than say that any of these foods are good or bad, I recognize that they help me feel a certain way. You may find you have the same reaction or you may need to experiment further and find what is most helpful to you in each context.

Right and Wrong

In a way, right and wrong takes us back to "should" and "shouldn't," and to expectations. When we think it's right to eat certain foods, behave in a particular way, or do certain things, we adopt a kind of mental rigidity. Once we have a concept of right and wrong that we apply to everyone, we then open ourselves to disappointment and frustration as other people, nations, religions, cultures, and societies will not necessarily adhere to our interpretations of right and wrong. I've noticed that even very small differences in the interpretation of right and wrong among family members can cause great upsets.

Our ideas on right and wrong tend to reflect our current cultures, societies, and chosen religions or spiritual beliefs. These are often learned and come from our parents, teachers, and peers. This is different from something that feels right to us, which comes from our intuition and our souls. These feelings are unique to us. It is these feelings that we can use to create our own ethics and morality.

I've noticed that people have a tendency to take the desire to live in a world of right and wrong from a social structure or religion, and transplant it into a subject like macrobiotics. On one level, this is fine—if you want to apply the right-and-wrong structure to food, exercise, and lifestyle. But you would also miss the opportunity to jump out of that way of thinking altogether, and experience life free from those set tracks.

It can also set us up for feelings of guilt if we think of eating bad foods as some kind of sin or failure. Once this happens, I think that the feeling of guilt is more harmful than the "bad" food.

JUDGMENTS

Another way we can fall into making assumptions is when we judge people. This might be a natural human response for trying to work out who is safe to be around and who we can trust, but it can also lead us to become disconnected from people. We will look at the effects of that disconnection in Chapter Eighteen.

Being judgmental can come from wanting to be part of a tribe, from wanting to know who are the good guys and bad guys are, and from a desire to elevate ourselves through putting someone else down. I went through a phase of wanting to be part of the macrobiotic tribe, and I also went through a phase of feeling superior to friends who were eating what I considered to be junk food. Looking back, I withdrew from these friends and disconnected myself. I now realize that if I had remained in a self-loving state I would not have felt superior, and I would have been able extend my love to those people who had been close to me. Fortunately, I came through that phase, but I recognize that it had a negative effect on me.

LETTING GO

The more time we can spend living in the moment, and living our lives as they happen, the easier it is to just live without getting caught up in what is right or wrong. When I'm feeling the sun, wind, or earth against my skin, there's no right or wrong. Similarly, when I relax and just feel my breath gently I feel completely free from any learned ideas of right and wrong.

Curiosity, desire to explore, enthusiasm to discover, and openness to revelations can all take us out of fixed views of right and wrong or good and bad. In my experience, I recognize that if I get caught up in my thoughts it's easier to slip back into being judgmental. It's when I am in my heart that I feel free to connect with other people and nature without thoughts of what should and shouldn't happen getting in the way.

For some people, letting go has come through the study of philosophy, engaging in Buddhist activities, taking up Taoist thought, or practicing meditation. The opportunities are everywhere; you may also find that art, poetry, music, writing, and crafts help you let go and just be.

For me, the most helpful has been to simply practice meditating on my breathing regularly.

PRACTICAL EXERCISES

1. Be aware of when you are thinking in terms of good and bad or right and wrong, or being judgmental. Catch yourself and make a mental note each time. This in itself can help you, as ideas get programmed into our subconscious and become a pattern of behavior.
2. When think in terms of good and bad or right and wrong remind yourself that this is a learned behavior and a choice. You don't have to think this way.

3. When you find yourself thinking in terms of good and bad or right and wrong, ask yourself how you feel. What are the effects of thinking this way?

4. Make time in every day to relax, be still, and feel your breathing. Gently start each in and out breath. As you feel more centered and better able to listen to your heart, see how you feel about things.

SUMMARY

1. Having beliefs in what is good or bad and right or wrong can limit our options. If we believe our interpretations of what is good or bad, right or wrong, is a universal truth, we risk loosing our connections with reality.

2. Rather than think in absolute terms of what is good or bad, it would be more realistic to think of how something like a food affects us without expecting it to have the same effect on everyone else all the time.

3. Thinking in terms of right and wrong sets up moral expectations that risk negative emotions.

4. Being judgmental of other people increases the risk of becoming disconnected from them, which can sabotage our healing processes.

5. Living in the moment and being in a still, self-loving state allows us to experience life without fixed ideas.

CHAPTER TEN

Emptying the Mind

The promise of macrobiotics is relief from an imbalanced state and coming to a sense of wellness. Well-being is a subjective indicator of health not quantified by medical testing. Contemplating symptoms of illness is stressful, while progressively feeling better is a feasible goal that offers encouragement and a continuously uplifting state of mind. This in itself adds to the joy of feeling better. The success of macrobiotics, therefore, is always evident in how we feel, without relying on "fixing" an illness.

—SHELDON RICE, numerologist, life coach,
and author of *Getting to Know You: A Numerology Textbook*

One of the biggest challenges we have is to stop thinking. There can be so much going on in our heads from waking to sleep that the whole day is spent processing the thoughts that are spinning around there. This takes us out of our hearts and away from our souls. Sometimes our thoughts can be negative and introduce emotions that are not helpful in terms of healing.

I used to try to consciously empty my mind while meditating. I was not successful with this approach, and found that it was easier to empty my mind by focusing on something simple. This worked well with a repetitive action that I was already familiar with. Breathing is the most obvious, as we are all used to breathing; however, an object of focus could be anything that we can do with very little thought.

Ultimately you'll find you can get into a state where you actually feel your soul and, from there, be able to connect with the love inside you. The more often you reach this state, the stronger the part of your brain that controls your emotions becomes. After a while you'll find that when you feel upset, all you have to do is go back to your breathing to get back to feeling calm.

FOCUSING ON REPETITIVE TASKS

Take a simple function that you can you do repetitively, such as riding a bicycle, ironing, or walking, and use this as the basis for emptying your mind. Take your chosen task and focus your mind on the action. If you're walking, be aware of the feeling of your heel making contact with the ground, your weight rolling onto the ball of your foot, and your toes bending as you lift your foot. If you can lose yourself in the feeling of walking, for the time you're doing it, you'll free your mind of all the thoughts that would normally whiz around in your head. I suggest using a task you are so familiar with, something you can do using your subconscious, so that you do not need to use your conscious mind to perform the task.

OBSERVATION

Another way to step out of our usual flow of thoughts is to find something to look at that you can ask questions of and lose yourself in your observations. This kind of meditation is summed up in the philosophy of *wabi sabi*. You could meditate by looking at a leaf, a twig, a candle flame, blistering paint, rotting driftwood, stained paper, frayed cloth, or a weathered stone. It can help if you find something that has aged, as this will give you another dimension to consider.

Start by looking at the object and carefully noting its color, shape, texture, shading, and how it has aged. Stare at the object and start asking questions: What does it look like, how was it formed, where did it come from, what does it remind you of, how do you feel about it?

BREATHING

Take a few seconds now to try this breathing meditation. Start by breathing gently, starting each in and out breath with your mind. Let the rest of your breath take its natural course. Do not force it or try to control your breath. Once you're comfortable starting each in and out breath, be aware of all the feelings of breathing. Feel the air in your nose and throat, be aware of the movement of your chest, notice the coolness of the air coming in and the warmth of the air leaving your body, experience any movement in your abdomen and any sense of your ribs accommodating your lungs.

FEELING

Take an object and feel it. You could roll some sand or a twig between your fingers, run your fingers over a stone or piece of wood, or walk barefoot over different surfaces. Try closing your eyes to focus solely on the feeling of the action on your skin.

You may find this good practice for touching another person. This meditation can help you feel someone's hair or skin and be totally in the moment of that feeling. You might be surprised at how this changes the experience for the other person.

LISTENING

Try listening to music or sounds in nature and being totally absorbed in each part of that experience. Next time someone is telling you something, see if you can be completely absorbed in listening. Hear the tone of your friend's voice, the intonation, and the energy behind the words. Resist the temptation to think of a response, and just trust that you will know what to say when appropriate.

SMELLING

Some of our earliest memories come from smells. You can meditate on various smells by breathing in a scent and using it as a focus for your mind.

TASTING

When eating or drinking, you can use the sensation of taste to help you be in the moment. Keep the drink or food in your mouth for as long as possible so you can really taste every flavor. Try to savor every mouthful and really enjoy each different flavor and texture.

PRACTICAL EXERCISES

1. Try all the forms of meditation described above, as each will strengthen a specific aspect of your senses.
2. You may find that you naturally prefer one type of meditation; this can become the meditation you return to in times of stress and emotional disturbance.
3. Try to stretch yourself so that you can meditate for longer periods. You might find it helps to time yourself. To begin with, see if you can become absorbed in your meditation for ten seconds; work your way up to a minute.
4. It helps to meditate several times a day and to practice in all types of environments. There is no need to be in a special place. I like to practice my gentle breathing on buses and trains, in cafés, and at home, as well as while sitting in the park and walking through the woods.

SUMMARY

1. Emptying our minds frees us from unnecessary thoughts and creates a calm where we can relax and better connect with our souls.
2. One way to empty our minds is to focus on a task we could almost do in our sleep. By being aware of doing a simple repetitive task, we can focus our thoughts on that simple action.
3. We can also focus our minds through being aware of our breathing, as well as through observation, touching, listening, smelling, and tasting.

CHAPTER ELEVEN
Continuous Transformation

Language is the house of Being. In its home man dwells. Those who think and those who create with words are the guardians of this home.

—MARTIN HEIDEGGER, German philosopher

Most everything carries baggage. That is, there almost always exists *a priori* (before the fact) an already-listening or preconception about the matter at hand, whatever that might be at any given time. That generally holds true whether we are talking about people, events, or, for example, a social movement such as macrobiotics. We exist in an already-knowing.

Thus, we must strip away some common misconceptions about macrobiotics, such as that it is primarily a dietary regimen. In fact, most macrobiotic practitioners would probably agree that it has something to do with diet. That is how ingrained the idea has become.

I would like to propose the radical idea that macrobiotics has nothing to do with practicing a diet. Now, a great deal of attention is brought to bear on food and its means of preparation, which we call cooking. No question about that. In macrobiotics we see the act of eating as the mediating process by which the outer world in the form of solids (food), liquids, air, light, sound, thoughts, information, etc. are internalized and become us. Literally, we eat the world and thus in a way are created by the world, one could say.

The reverse is true as well, we could say. As soon as we open our mouths and begin to speak—or even think, for that matter—we are creating the world by means of language or through our interpretations of what or who is out there. There is no world, per se, other than the one given by the model of reality or paradigm in which we're living at any given time. Literally, we create the world and each other every time we open our mouths.

Macrobiotics at its essence, I would venture, is about awakening to the mutually constitutive (distinct but not separate) relationship we have with the world and what it means and where it's going.

—GREG JOHNSON, teacher, facilitator, and director of the Community Health Foundation, London

A CLEARING FOR POSSIBILITY

One of George Ohsawa's basic claims was that everything changes. This thought can be found in Taoism, Zen Buddhism, and *wabi sabi* as well as in modern science. The world we live in is in a state of change, and we are changing with it. In science, it's said that the only constant is change. The message is that if we cling to the same beliefs and thoughts for too long, we risk being out of harmony with the world around us and even out of harmony with ourselves.

I like to think of this as a continual path of transformation. One of the abilities we are rarely taught is how to transform ourselves. Looking back over my life, I can see that I would happily stay in modes of behavior while my life was going well and only engage in change when faced with difficulties. It was as though I would let myself become static, slowly becoming further disconnected from my changing world and self until being shocked into having to catch up. Unfortunately, it has taken separation, divorce, financial difficulties, and minor health issues to jolt me out of my complacency. It has only been recently that I have embraced transformation without a strong and obvious stimulus.

One of the greatest blocks to deep transformation is taking the easy option of transferring to another belief system. You'll know this is happening if you're switching from one guru or subject to another. The risk of this is that only techniques and methods change, and deeper things remain stuck.

For me, transformation happens best when I can put all my beliefs to one side. When I can let go of other people's amazing insights and theories for a while. This is when I am naked with myself. I am most exposed and best able to connect with my deeper self and experience real change.

Greg Johnson claims that big block to transformation is hope. Hope lulls us into feeling that one day it will all work out even if we don't change. Hope becomes an excuse for hiding from transformation. Serge Benhayon says the belief that everything happens for a reason keeps us away from connecting with our souls and embracing change.

PARADIGM SHIFTS

Humans have gone through extraordinary shifts in thinking. These are known as paradigm shifts. We once thought our world was flat; then we thought it was round, with our sun revolving around us. We finally moved on to thinking that we are a speck on the edge of an expanding universe. Each phase brought a different perception of ourselves and our relationship with our universe. Humans in each phase thought that their perception was the final version, and many people think our current interpretation of how the universe works—with particles, atoms, and molecules—is the final version, and would be amazed to think there may be a whole new interpretation around the corner. Human history has witnessed Newtonian mechanical physics; Einstein's theories of relativity; and, later, quantum physics, where instead of rules, we have a world defined by probabilities. Again there have been shifts in our relationship to our world as a result of each paradigm shift.

Similarly, macrobiotics has been through many big shifts. To take just the recent history, there has been Sagen Ishizuka's approach to eating natural foods in season while exploring the acidity and alkalinity, and sodium-potassium ratios; George Ohsawa's philosophical approach; and Michio Kushi's standard diet, Asian medicine, and principles. Now it is changing to be more holistic, intuitive, and open to working with our hearts and emotions.

We will inevitably go through more amazing paradigm shifts, and our relationship with everything around us will keep changing. The point here is not to be attached to any one part of this process.

HAVING A FEEDBACK SYSTEM

In his book *Psycho-Cybernetics,* Maxwell Maltz talks about having a feedback system. He likens human development to a rocket. The rocket recognizes when it is off-course through its feedback system, and makes adjustments. Having adjusted its course, it will start to go off-course again, recognize this, and make further adjustments. If we don't have a feedback system we can drift further and further off-course and never realize it.

Part of the awareness for recognizing whether we are off-course, off-balance, or out of harmony comes from self-reflection. Again, I have found it easiest to use my gentle breathing meditation as a measure of my current state. If I find it hard to let go of thoughts and emotions and slip into feeling still and centered, I know I have become disconnected or lost some of my harmony with nature. My dreams, sleep, bowel movements, skin, emotions, moods, energy levels, and mental clarity can all provide feedback on my current state. These are explored in greater detail in Chapter Twenty-One, "Testing Our Bodies." This helps me be aware and engage in a continuous process of transformation.

Learning from Experience

One of the biggest teachers in life is experience. We can read books, go to lectures, and watch films to learn how to ride a bike, but in the end we will learn only through actually getting on a bike, falling off, trying again, falling off, and trying again until we manage to balance, steer, and peddle all the same time.

One of the drawbacks of modern society is that we're generally not encouraged to learn from our mistakes. Our school systems, home lives, and work lives are generally set up to reward us when we do something that is considered correct and retrain us when we do something that is considered a mistake. We are therefore conditioned to learn something and to try and follow it without making mistakes. This methodology runs through many new age, complementary therapies. Even something like holistic massage is taught so that the masseuse learns to follow a set procedure and is discouraged from trying something different. Macrobiotic cooking has been taught in the same way.

To learn from experience, we need to celebrate mistakes. Mistakes are necessary for any learning to happen. This is particularly relevant to macrobiotics, where ideally each person would feel free to experiment, make mistakes, learn, make adjustments, and try again. It's only when we give ourselves the freedom and have the courage to make mistakes that we can really engage in transformation.

On a deeper level, I could question whether there really are such things as mistakes. Perhaps what we think of as mistakes are really artificially defined by society, and in that sense illusions that block our growth.

Honesty

Without honesty, there can be no accurate feedback system. If our feedback becomes corrupted through, for example, wishful thinking and the desire to cover up our perceived failings, we risk misleading ourselves and throwing ourselves further from our centers and feelings of harmony. Without honesty it would be hard to make mistakes and learn from them. Without honesty, we might not even admit to our mistakes or recognize them.

Honesty is the key to transformation, as without it we're simply playing with our delusions: messing around with things we made up in our heads. To make one big transformational change, start by practicing being honest with yourself. Once we can be honest with ourselves, we can begin to be honest with other people.

STILLNESS

Sometimes transformation can come out of disaster, stress, hopelessness, near-death experiences, and extreme emotions; however, there is a risk that in such drama the transformation will be unpredictable. It's more likely that when our energies are stirred up, we become disconnected from our souls and lose our intuition. Transformation can also come out of stillness. There are times in life when we reach such a stillness that we can access our deepest feelings and, through that, experience life-changing revelations. In my experience, this happens most easily through gentle breathing and meditation. However, my ability to find a deep stillness can be enhanced by eating a diet high in vegetables, grains, beans, and fruit. It is much harder to find that stillness while consuming stimulants in the form of alcohol, coffee, sugar, chocolate, drugs, cigarettes, and strong spices.

In addition, different times of day might work better for some people. Getting up early and meditating while the sun rises over the horizon may help one person; for another it might be best to sit under the stars on a clear night. Some people find it easier to feel still around the new moon. You might also find that certain locations help you feel better able to experience your stillness. Sometimes large, airy buildings such as cathedrals make it easier. Sometimes being in nature helps—sitting under a willow tree next to a river, looking out over a moonlit sea, or standing on the top of a mountain. The more we practice, the stronger our connections become and the less important exterior influences are.

PRACTICAL EXERCISES

1. Write out a page on how you have changed though your life. Think about how your views have evolved since childhood. Write out any changes you have experienced in your health. Use this to remind yourself that further changes will happen.

2. Make a list of elements that could form part of your feedback system. For example, you might include dreams, sleep, bowel movements, skin condition, emotions, moods, energy levels, and mental clarity. Write out honestly your experience of each. There is no need to interpret or look for answers. The aim is to simply have a feedback system. So you might write: "I have nightmares about drowning, I often wake at 4 a.m., I have a bowel movement every other day, my skin erupts after sugary foods, I get irritable when tired, I am prone to depression, I get tired in the afternoon, and I lose concentration after meals."

3. Write out mistakes you've made and what you've learned from them. If you can't think of any, try being more adventurous with your life!

4. Make an honest list of aspects of yourself you would like to change. You might need to do this in your head a few times before having the courage to commit to writing these aspects down on paper.

5. Try your gentle breathing meditation after consuming alcohol, coffee, sugar, chocolate, drugs, cigarettes, or strong spices to feel the difference for yourself. I find it best to go for a few weeks without indulging in any

of those substances, and to then try something like a strong coffee and, after an hour, experiment with my meditation.

6. Try eating natural, whole foods for a few days and be aware of any changes in the ease with which you feel a deep stillness.

7. Experiment with the gentle breathing meditation at different times of day and in different places to see if you notice any consistent influences.

SUMMARY

1. George Ohsawa embedded the premise that everything changes into macrobiotic philosophy.

2. There have been huge shifts in human awareness, known as paradigm shifts, that have brought about huge changes in our relationship with the world around us. Macrobiotics has and is also in a process of change. Whatever we believe makes up macrobiotics will evolve and change over time.

3. Humans need an accurate, real, and honest feedback system to guide us through transformation.

4. Making mistakes is one way of learning from experience.

5. Honesty is essential for accurate feedback.

6. In moments of stillness, we can access our souls and intuition to guide us through our processes of transformation.

CHAPTER TWELVE
Nutrition for the Mind

Top Ten Things I've Learned from a Thirty-Five-Year Macrobiotics Practice

1. Never combine beans and fruit—unless you want to clear a room quickly.
2. It is possible to chew thoroughly on one side and talk from the other.
3. I am definitely not Japanese—gimme a fluffy bed and a four-legged table, and cook my fish, please.
4. Go easy on yin/yang terminology. It makes you sound like Confucius.
5. Always brush your teeth after eating seaweed—especially the black stringy varieties.
6. There's only one "should": you should never tell people what they should eat.
7. Believe your aunt when she says, "Seaweed makes me throw up."
8. Yes, walking barefoot on dewy grass is good—but not near dog parks.
9. Despite what you may read in macrobiotic cookbooks, tofu never tastes just like cheese.
10. Macrobiotic cats should not be on an exclusive brown mice diet.

—VERNE VARONA, macrobiotic teacher and counselor,
and author of *Nature's Cancer-Fighting Foods* and *Macrobiotics for Dummies*

George Ohsawa introduced the idea that our diets might influence our thinking and Michio Kushi expanded upon it. This even includes the proposition that different cultures think the way they do because of their natural diets. For example, a culture eating strong spicy foods might feel more stimulated and perhaps develop their thinking to be more imaginative, while a culture eating foods with more moderate tastes might be more functional.

It's a long-held view that eating fish helps increase intelligence. More recently, research suggests that schoolchildren consuming a wide range of vitamins and minerals can concentrate for longer. Research also indicates that when young schoolchildren don't have foods with added sugar, they tend to be less disruptive. My own experience has been that foods and drinks containing coffee, sugar, or chocolate are stimulating to my mind and help me come up with a wealth of ideas. If I'm writing in this state, I can write thousands of words in a short time. At the same time, my thinking becomes more chaotic and less focused. I also find that when I later read through a chapter written in a stimulated state, I have to rewrite much of it. More important, I would like to offer you something that comes from deeper within than a coffee-, sugar-, and chocolate-fueled mind.

For many years I've been aware of how my mind works after eating different foods, and I can choose which foods to eat when I want to use my mind in a certain way.

FOOD, BLOOD, AND THE BRAIN

One way that food affects our thinking is that whatever we eat has an influence on our blood, and our blood flows through our brains. If I were to eat a food that raised my blood sugar quickly, my brain would respond and I would find it easier to use my mind in a certain way. In my experience, this helps me think about lots of things at once and have more wild ideas. I am also aware that I find it harder to complete a train of thought without getting distracted.

The effect that people recognize most easily is feeling sleepy after eating a large meal with lots of saturated fats (such as fried eggs and/or meats, and cheese), as we try to digest the food and our blood becomes richer in fats for a while.

A lack of minerals and vitamins is thought to affect our concentration and, conversely, studies indicate that children who eat more mineral- and vitamin-rich foods are better able to concentrate for longer periods. Poor concentration is made worse when refined sugar is added to the diet. There is also speculation that eating modern processed soy foods (this does not include fermented soy foods—miso, shoyu, natto, and tempeh) increases the risk of premature brain-related degenerative illness such as Alzheimer's disease.

I would suggest that for ideal long-term mental health, explore eating a wide range of mineral- and vitamin-rich foods. This could include vegetables, fish, beans, grains, fruits, nuts, seeds, and fermented foods. To build up knowledge of your own relationship between food and thinking, it's important to experiment. To gain valuable experience, you'll need to eat a wide variety of foods and be aware of how well you can use your mind before and after eating.

THE ENERGY OF FOODS

In macrobiotic thinking, we also consider foods to have a life force, also described as living energy. The idea is that the living energy of each food we eat will influence our own energies. The states of our energies then have an effect on our thinking. My aim here is to help you think about another dimension to eating, and start to develop your own awareness. These are not rules, but my own experiences and those of other people in the macrobiotics movement; I hope they will inspire you to play with the idea that whatever you put in your mouth may have a subtle influence on how you use your mind. The information here can provide an entry point for your journey of discovering how food influences you. You can read more about the energy of foods in Chapter Thirty-One.

In my experience, the effects of food on thinking are subtle, and you may need to eat a certain food for some time before being aware of its influence. All people will experience the energy of foods in their own way, and therefore writing about the energy of foods is a big generalization. The foods that help me feel calm might lead to someone else feeling dull; the foods I like to eat to feel more creative might lead to feelings of impatience in another person.

You could experiment with looking at any food you're eating and seeing if you can intuitively feel what kind of effect it will have on your mind. For example, a large fresh salad might have a cooling effect on your mind and help you think clearly and make a decision, whereas a bowl of hot noodles in broth might spread a feeling of warmth to your head, helping you relax and absorb ideas.

In macrobiotic theory, foods that grow upwards—like green vegetables—have more of an up energy. These would be more cooling to our minds and send a more "up" feeling to our heads than, say, a root vegetable soup, which has more of a warming influence and also has as its ingredients vegetables that grow down into the ground. The soup could have a more grounding influence, helping us think in more practical terms, while steamed greens could help us have more inspiring ideas.

Some dishes will bring a faster energy to our beings. Quickly stir-fried and mildly spicy vegetables can bring a rush of energy into our minds, perhaps stimulating our creativity for a while.

It is also interesting to experiment with eating animal foods and seeing whether the character and nature of the animal carries through into our thinking. Does eating salmon, for example, help us metaphorically swim upstream and express thoughts that go against the grain of society? How does that feeling compare with eating mackerel or herring, which swim in schools and move together? Is eating beef better for feeling calm than eating a relatively lively animal like chicken?

Perhaps the biggest question is whether eating a seed-based diet, with lots of seeds, nuts, dried beans, and whole grains, means that by consuming foods with a very young energy, ready to grow into a plant, results in us being more open-minded and ready to explore new ideas. Also, is the opposite true? Does eating mature, fully grown foods such as meat, fish, and vegetables help us think in a way that is less naive and more competitive and streetwise?

We could also try eating primitive foods like sea vegetables (wakame, nori, kombu, arame, dulse), shellfish (mussels, clams, oysters, snails), and fermented foods (miso, shoyu, sauerkraut, vinegars, pickles) and see if this primal energy helps us think about the more primitive aspects of life: sex and survival.

PRACTICAL EXERCISES

1. Experiment by avoiding all coffee, alcohol, sugar, strong spices, and chocolate for one week and see how this influences your thinking.
2. Try not eating foods high in saturated fats for one week and see if you notice a difference in your mind. Foods high in saturated fats are meats, eggs, poultry, cheese, milk, butter, and yogurt. Instead, you could eat more fish, seafood, hummus, tahini, tofu, beans, olive oil, and nuts.

3. Make an effort to increase your consumption of a variety of vegetables (for example, carrots, broccoli, radishes, cauliflower, onions, watercress, parsley, leafy greens, pumpkin, and scallions), fruits (such as apples, pears, berries, apricots, melon, and grapes), nuts (almonds, hazelnuts, walnuts, peanuts), seeds (sunflower, pumpkin, sesame), and fish for one week, while also reducing your sugar intake, to see if you become aware of a change in your ability to concentrate.

4. Spend a day eating mainly vegetables that grow upwards (such as broccoli, greens, scallions, cauliflower, herbs) and be aware of how your mind feels.

5. Eat a meal consisting of stir-fried vegetables with spices (garlic, ginger, wasabi, mustard, or chilies) and, if you wish, grains (leftover brown rice or precooked noodles); be aware of your thinking an hour or two later.

6. Try eating one kind of fish or meat for a few weeks and see if you notice any change in your thinking. Does the change you experience reflect any aspect of the character of the animal?

7. Introduce miso soups, pickles, sauerkraut, sea vegetable salad, clams, mussels, oysters, and a little shoyu into your diet and be aware of any tendency toward more primal thoughts and desires for sex.

SUMMARY

1. The macrobiotic view is that our diets can affect our thinking.
2. Studies of children indicate that good nutrition and an absence of added sugar increase concentration.
3. Including fish in our diets is thought to improve intelligence.
4. Stimulants like coffee, sugar, strong spices, alcohol, and chocolate can alter our thinking.
5. A meal high in saturated fats can lead to a sleepy mind.
6. Modern processed soy foods such as soy milk, yogurt, cheese, spreads, and sausages may increase the risk of degenerative brain disease.
7. Leafy greens and vegetables that grow upward can subtly help us be clear minded.

8. Well-cooked root vegetables can make it subtly easier to think in practical terms.

9. Dishes cooked quickly over a high flame, such as stir fries, can help us feel a little more mentally active for a while.

10. Eating foods that are at the beginning of their lives, such as grains, bean, nuts, and seeds, may help us be inclined to take on new ideas and explore new subjects.

11. Eating fish, meat, and vegetables (which are at the end of their lives) can encourage us to be more competitive.

12. Primitive foods such as sea vegetables, fermented foods, and shellfish may encourage us to think more about our primal desires for sex and survival.

PART THREE
HEALING THE HEART

In this section, I will take you on a journey though the macrobiotic practices that come together and help us heal our hearts. Here you will explore your emotions, love, and feelings.

You will discover ways to free yourself from unwanted emotions and find an entrance to self-love, love, and appreciation. This can become a powerful home and center for your healing journey in life. We will also explore the ultimate expression of macrobiotics and how we nurture our souls during this life.

We will work through different practical exercises to feel our emotional bodies and work with those emotions. In addition, we will discuss the role of food and other influences on our energetic bodies.

CHAPTER THIRTEEN
Listening to Our Emotions

A true healing can only come from your soul. The soul heals the spirit, by choice when it is willing or by necessity when it has caused too much harm to the self and also too others. The soul heals by reducing and or arresting the excessive *prana,* or by transmuting the stagnated energy that the human spirit operates in.

When it comes to healing, there are many pitfalls, for many think or believe that healing is curing when the two are not energetically one and the same.

This does not mean that true miracles cannot occur, or that a cure cannot also be a healing; it does, however, inspire one to contemplate deeply the fact that all is not what it seems and therefore, a reliance on results, and or experience, leaves one naught in true truth, if the energy of the experience is not truly known.

—SERGE BENHAYON, esoteric healer, teacher, and author

Humans have an emotional body and an emotional intelligence. Some people consider the heart to have an intelligence of its own. Our emotional bodies work through an energy, or life force, that runs through everything in the universe. In a way, we can feel emotionally connected to everything else. This connection does not mean we lose our ability to create our own emotions—far from it. We have a choice over how we feel, and it enables us to feel empathy, compassion, and an emotional bond with everything we know.

Sometimes we shut out our emotions because to experience them is painful, and we go into emotional denial. Although this is understandable, it also stops our development and prevents us from working with difficult emotions as part of a process of healing. In my experience, it's easier to heal when I allow even the most painful emotions to remain alive in me, when I move them and play with them rather than suppress or bury them. Once pushed deep inside and left there, they can contribute to an unhealthy stagnation in our energetic bodies.

The first step to working with our emotional bodies is to be aware of them. As you might guess having read this book so far, the way to access our emotions is to turn off our minds for a while so that we can feel instead of think.

LIE DOWN AND RELAX

One way to listen to your emotions is to feel your body. To you do this, I suggest you simply get used to listening to your body. Try not to judge yourself, make excuses, or add meaning to what you feel. The only objective to this exercise is to feel each part of your body.

Lie down on a bed, sofa, or floor and make yourself comfortable. Start with your abdomen and chest: start to think about how you feel there emotionally. Do you feel any anxiety? Is there a tightness in your stomach due to stress? Do you feel a sense of frustration across your middle? Does your chest feel tight, and do you feel that you have suppressed emotions there? Are there any places that feel empty and sad? Does your heart feel calm with a relaxed pulse? Where do you feel calm? Can you access a feeling of love? Do you feel content? Can you experience a feeling of self-belief?

Try this exercise every day to get a feel for how you are and how you change from one day to the next. As you do this, you'll become more aware of your feelings and better able to identify how you are emotionally. It is only through feeling and acknowledging our emotions that we can work with them.

GENTLE BREATHING

It can be the case that our minds introduce thinking that is judgmental, makes comparisons between us and other people, and introduces expectations that increase the pain we feel when we access certain emotions. It is only when we turn our minds off from this thinking through breathing meditation that we can work with our emotional bodies without having distressing thoughts flood in.

Going into our gentle breathing meditations, we reach a state where it is safe to experience our emotional bodies. Simply breathing gently, initiating each breath, and focusing on the feel of each breath is enough to prevent our minds from bringing distressing learned responses to our emotional bodies. I find that in this state I can experience and be aware of my emotions without feeling pain. This is a vital step in listening to our emotions, as once we are able to experience them without pain we can open up to being aware of emotions that have been buried for a long time. These emotions likely have been buried long ago because of our fears that they would be too distressing to work with. Again, I would like to acknowledge and thank Serge Benhayon for introducing me to this experience.

PRACTICAL EXERCISES

1. Practice listening to your body.
2. Be aware how different parts of your body feel and whether there are any emotions associated with parts of your body.
3. Practice your gentle breathing meditation.
4. Once in a peaceful state, and while focused on your breathing, allow emotions to surface naturally.
5. Rest with your emotions and get used being with them.

SUMMARY

1. We have emotional bodies, but they can be masked by our minds.
2. When we switch off our minds, we become more aware of our emotional bodies.
3. One way to begin to be more aware of our emotional bodies is to practice feeling our physical bodies.
4. We may find in the process of feeling our bodies that some parts of our bodies hold certain emotions.
5. We sometimes suppress painful emotions, pushing the energy of those emotions deeper into our bodies.

6. When we meditate on our breathing, we can access our deeper emotions without our minds bringing painful thoughts.

7. In this state we can let deep emotions from the past surface freely and accept them as they are.

CHAPTER FOURTEEN
Endless Appreciation and Love

Macrobiotics has allowed me to realize that even seemingly insurmount-able issues can be seen in the "big view." We are all free to play, to dream, and to go our own way, yet when we acknowledge the real suffering of others, growing world hunger, violent conflicts, delusions of fanaticism and the future we leave to the next generation, why would anyone choose to escape?

In the spirit of one grain to ten thousand grains, I am first responsible for my own health, while recognizing there is really only one of us here—one human family. Freedom is ultimately born out of transcending a self-centered existence, accepting that the world is perfect right now—and that there's plenty more we can do to make it better. I'm all in.

—WILLIAM SPEAR, author of *Feng Shui Made Easy* and *Recovering Original Ability*,
macrobiotic teacher, counselor, feng shui consultant, and guide

Inside our bodies are our souls, and our souls know only love. When we access and feel our souls, we feel love. We feel love of ourselves and a love of everything. George Ohsawa expressed it as appreciation, and talked about having an endless appreciation for life.

These feelings produce far-reaching changes throughout our bodies, and they go on to change our relationships with everything around us. People react differently when we express love, the world appears differently when we see it through love, and even our food tastes different when we cook and eat with love.

You might ask, Why we are not like this all the time? Unfortunately, we shroud these beautiful feelings in layers of beliefs, ideologies, behavioral patterns, habits, assumptions, judgments, and our successful coping strategies. I would suggest that what we think of as our personalities and characters are actually masks covering the warmth and light that emanate from our souls.

APPRECIATION

Research on the DNA helix shows that when it is surrounded by actors generating feelings of anger, it contracts; it becomes most expanded when the actors generate feelings of appreciation.

I would recommend that we start by appreciating ourselves first and then see where that takes us in terms of appreciating life as a whole. In my experience, at times when I have felt self-loathing, I have not been able to appreciate anything else.

Whatever our situations, we can deeply appreciate ourselves. We are amazing creatures, and every human has much to wonder and love about him- or herself. Even in times of ill health, we can marvel at the way we can preserve physical life for as long as possible. Our bodies go to extraordinary lengths and perform extraordinary feats to keep us alive. The mere fact that we are still alive is something to appreciate and love about ourselves.

Often our bodies will try to move harmful substances toward the exterior. This may show up as problems with skin, breast lumps, hemorrhoids, mucus, changes in hair quality, abnormal menstruation, or various discharges. We may see these kinds of issues as a problem, but we could instead appreciate our bodies' ability to protect us from more serious problems.

Even at times of serious illness, we have amazing capacities to regenerate and heal. People have recovered from all kinds of cancers, even when the medical profession had given up. Our hearts can grow new arteries around one that is blocked, our livers will regenerate to compensate for chemical abuse, we have wisdom teeth ready to grow and move other teeth forward to fill in a gap resulting from serious decay.

More than that, each challenge can take us into new adventures that help us evolve. I personally went through a phase of change and growth after a divorce. I have also had to evolve during times of financial challenge. It's partly through these events that I've developed the resources I have; therefore, it would make sense for me to appreciate those challenges, even though they were painful at the time, for stimulating me to be more open to change. George Ohsawa even encouraged his students to go out and purposefully take on challenges so that they could grow.

If we choose, we can continually appreciate ourselves for being the amazing expressions of life that we are. We can choose to appreciate challenges for being the stimulus for change, for jump-starting us out of a period of stagnation. If we make this choice, we become beautiful in body, mind, and heart, and we're able to embrace our own healing.

LOVE

In my experience, love starts from our souls, and when we find our love, it radiates freely. We might first feel a love inside ourselves, and then out of that feel a love for everything we know. It is likely that this feeling is what the word "enlightenment" is used for. In terms of energy, love feels like a fire or light inside us. We could make association between the sun and love, the energy of fire and love, light and love. This is why the word is "en*light*enment."

Enlightenment has often been held up as something almost out of reach, difficult to attain; and yet, accessing the love in our souls is surprisingly easy. All we have to do is unwrap the layers of beliefs, concepts, constructs, judgments, assumptions, attachments, successful coping strategies, and habits of comparing ourselves to others that mask our souls. To manually try to take away each of these would be hard work and take a lifetime, but we can reach many moments of feeling love every day through our gentle breathing meditation.

I've found that the more time I spend living in a feeling of love, the more it spills over into everyday life. As this happens, my ego (the part of me that engages in self-obsession, feeling important, seeking admiration, creating a self-image, self-promotion, and feeling that it's all about me) dissolves naturally. In this state, it's much easier to let go and just be my true self.

Another way we can make it harder to feel our own love is when we give away our power to another person. If we become a follower of a guru, we take on his or her beliefs and ideals; by doing so, we create a strong barrier to connecting with our souls. In my humble opinion, this is one of the most disempowering aspects of the new age movement. It has meant that rather than freeing ourselves, we have simply switched from one set of beliefs to another, and from giving our selves away to one person to giving ourselves away to another. In this sense, some of the interpretations of new age beliefs mirror some of the interpretations of religious beliefs from the previous age.

As Dragana wrote in our macrobiotics Internet discussion group, education stems from the Latin word *educo,* translated as "to draw out." The true meaning of education could be said to be to draw out of ourselves that which is already inside us—to find our own truths rather have them imposed on us.

We might also become enslaved to certain principles, and once we feel attached to them it becomes harder to let go and be open to the feeling of love. This would even apply to many worthy causes. Veganism, vegetarianism, pacifism, environmentalist, social justice, and modes of healing (including macrobiotics) would all be examples that I would naturally sympathize with; however, once I believe in them and take them on as absolutes, I generate a mindset that becomes another layer surrounding my soul.

This is where the idea of non-credo comes in. If I feel like eating a vegan diet one day, I can do so without wrapping a mask around my soul. I may feel like it for many days or even a lifetime, I don't know. It's when I believe I *am* vegan that I create the mask. Similarly with macrobiotics, I prefer to feel it rather than think it. I generally eat what I feel like, but I eat with awareness and use each meal as part of my learning about food.

Once we feel the love radiating from our souls, it's interesting to find that it's universal. Love is not selective or judgmental or conditional. It is a universal feeling. I believe it is in those moments when you feel a universal love for everything that you are connected to your soul; in these moments you may discover many truths about yourself. You may have revelations, insights, and intuitive feelings that prove to be life-changing.

I would highly recommend experiencing macrobiotics while in a state of universal love, as it is then that you can feel your truth about food, health, and healing.

HEALING

To help connect with your soul and feel love, try the following: Lie on your back somewhere comfortable. Put a cushion under your head or neck and, if necessary under your knees.

Place one hand on your lower abdomen between your navel and your pubic bone. Place your other hand over the center of your chest, between your nipples. Relax and consciously initiate every in and out breath. Be aware of the feeling of breathing. Feel the movement in your nose, mouth, throat, chest, and abdomen.

After a minute or so you may feel your hands get hotter as energy flows between your hands and body. If you have managed to stay in the moment and clear your head of everything except your breathing, you will be ready to feel your love.

With a feeling of love and stillness you can create imaginary hands that can float into your body and cuddle different parts of your body. If you're aware of any cold areas inside, take your imaginary hands there to bring warmth and love.

If you feel comfortable working on yourself in this way, you can then do the same with another person. One person lies on his or her back, and the other places his or her hands on the chest and lower abdomen. It's fine to be wearing clothes, although I would suggest that pure cotton would be better than synthetic clothing. If the person lying down is female, be sensitive not to make contact with her breasts.

Both of you can then go into your gentle breathing meditation and just feel each breath. In this state, a loving energy will be free to pass between you. You may notice the palms of your hands getting hot as the fiery loving energy passes between you. If thoughts enter your mind, be aware of them and then return your awareness to your breathing.

PRACTICAL EXERCISES

1. Thank yourself for being the wonderful expression of life that you are.
2. Thank yourself for keeping you alive so far.

3. Try to cultivate a deep sense of appreciation, wonder, and marvel for being the person you are. Think of the millions of years it has taken to evolve a creature that's as wonderful as you.

4. Study the human body, research the mind, and explore the emotional body so that you can appreciate the extraordinary splendor that we all are.

5. Consider a health problem you've had. Try to understand the healing process your body went through. If you currently have a health issue, explore the ways your body is working to preserve your life.

6. Go back through your life and note any big challenge you faced. Write out how you responded to this challenge, and how you've evolved as a result.

7. Write out a list of beliefs you have. Think about whether you would lose anything by not having those beliefs.

8. Make a list of people whose ideas have a strong influence on you. This could include teachers, gurus, family members, friends, writers, or colleagues. Think about your relationship with each person, and consider whether you are making it harder to find your own truth through this interaction.

9. Write out any principles you feel strongly about. Think about how you could put them to one side and live in the moment. Note that the more attached you are to something, the greater a layer it makes around your soul.

10. Practice your gentle breathing meditation every day, and strengthen your connection to your soul.

11. Place your hands over your chest and abdomen while initiating every in and out breath and being aware of your breathing.

12. Take your imaginary hands inside your body and love, cuddle, and hug each part of yourself.

SUMMARY

1. Our souls know only love.
2. The world is different to us when we are in a state of love.
3. We tend to hide our souls under layers of beliefs, ideologies, behavior patterns, habits, assumptions, judgments, and our successful coping strategies.
4. Our DNA expands when we feel appreciation.
5. Appreciating ourselves, whether in health or sickness, is important for healing.
6. Every challenge is an opportunity to grow, and we can approach each challenge with a feeling of appreciation.
7. To feel universal love is easy and possible in a short space of time.
8. By experiencing our breathing meditations every day, we can begin to connect with our souls and feel love. In this state our egos slip away more easily, helping us let go of beliefs and attachments.
9. We may give our power away to another person or guru and, by doing so, dissipate our connections to our own souls and to love.
10. We can become enslaved to other people's ideas, beliefs, or principles and thereby, lose our own truths and connections to our love.
11. Love is universal—not selective, conditional, or judgmental.

CHAPTER FIFTEEN
Opening Your Heart

Macrobiotics is infinite life itself, and everyone is macrobiotic, whether or not they say so. Practicing macrobiotics is to participate in the process of consciously transforming, creating ourselves. Utilizing the universal principles of polarity and mastering the art of change enables us to change sickness and suffering into well-being and happiness. And diet, which originally meant "way of life," is really eating infinity in all its myriad forms, adapting to an ever-changing environment. This makes macrobiotics the consummate adventure, wonderful and awesome—a veritable heaven on earth!

—BOB CARR, macrobiotic teacher and counselor

The heart and chest area is often the location where we feel our strongest emotions; it's where we feel love emanate from. The heart area has a special role in healing, as it is here that we can balance our bodies and minds. Simply opening the heart to create a freer flow of energy between our bodies and minds can be healing in itself.

It's easy for us to shut down the energy around our hearts through disappointments, rejection, lack of love, and abandonment. This can easily happen in childhood, while we are still forming our physical and energetic bodies. It could also happen later, through traumas at school, rejection in love, or the death of someone close.

Once the heart energy becomes constricted, it can be harder for our energies, or life forces, to flow between our bodies and minds. This can lead to feeling disconnected. It feels as though we have ideas, and we have feelings—but the two are separate. Once our hearts open and our energies move freely, we can feel our thoughts in our body and have a greater mental awareness of what's happening in our bodies. Ultimately, this allows our intuition to work fully and on all levels. We become whole—and our bodies and minds work together as one. Out of this, our intuition may become more apparent.

CHAKRAS

In the Indian view of the human energy body, there are seven energy centers known as chakras. These are places where there is an increased activity in our life forces and emotional energies. The heart chakra is the central energy center. Its position is midway between the more physical chakras, concerned with reproduction, power, and will, and those that are more mental, relating to communication, intellect, and spirit.

You could think of the heart energy center as being between the instinctive energy of our reproductive organs, intestines, and stomach and the intellectual energy of our throat, mind, and crown. In this theory, our hearts are the balancing and mixing point. Our hearts form an energetic channel between the body and mind. When it's closed, and we feel a separation between body and mind; when it's open, we feel whole and complete.

I found that when I started to explore macrobiotics in my twenties I did so in a highly intellectual way; I now realize my heart chakra felt constricted at that time. I was not aware of it, as I didn't know any different. It was only later that I really experienced the difference. Once my heart opened up I could feel macrobiotics, and my relationships with people took on a new dimension; I could connect with stronger emotions.

MAKING LOVE

It is said of chakras that when they are all, open energy flows freely through and we get a glimpse of divinity. Some people spend their whole lives chanting, meditating, and adopting special physical stances to try to open all their chakras at the same time.

Nature has created a natural means to experience this through lovemaking. When two people make love (in my experience, with love and not simply mechanical sex), we can experience the kind of orgasm that opens all our chakras, letting energy rush through all the energy centers, from the ones behind our pubic bones to the ones at the top of our heads. It may be that in that divine state we can accept our Gods and the creation of new lives into our beings. Next time you're able to make love with someone, do so with an awareness of how you feel in all these places.

Women appear to experience this more strongly. According to the women I have talked to, the energy starts in the heart and moves through the abdomen to behind the pubic bone. Kissing stimulates the throat chakra. Feelings of love can rise up through the mind to the top of the head or crown. When all these seven energy centers are open and stimulated, then an orgasm allows energy to surge through all the centers at the same time. In males, it may work in the opposite way: starting in the mind and pubic area, working inward to the heart chakra. Ultimately the same experience can occur where all the energy centers open. When this occurs, in both sexes there is a moment of surrender as we let go of our conscious minds and slip into pure energy. This has a slight similarity to when we fall asleep. (It's also possible that this feeling of surrender is something we experience when we are ready to leave our bodies.) You might find that approaching the moment of orgasm with gentleness helps you experience it more fully and for longer.

SOUL

The heart chakra is considered not only to be the center of our emotional bodies, but also part of the location of our souls. It is through connecting with this emotional center that we can feel our intuition, find our truths, and use them to make choices about food, exercise, spiritual practices, and life in general. This is where you might find the real you. It's what's left when we strip out all our beliefs, concepts, constructs, assumptions, judgments, shoulds, and shouldn'ts.

You might find a feeling of purity and clarity here that can give you wonderful insights and revelations. More important, it is when the heart chakra opens that we experience universal and unconditional love. As I have written earlier, it is out of this feeling that we can take on change and transformation.

My experience has been that initially I enjoyed only glimpses of being in my heart and soul and feeling universal love. These might occur for a few seconds here or there in a day. As time went by, I could generate this feeling for longer and experience it more often. Then the feeling would tend to spill over into general life.

When I am in this feeling, it's harder to do myself harm by eating foods that I like but have found not to be good for me.

To help open this area, be aware of your posture. Try to avoid slouching; sit or stand in a way that makes your heart relaxed but open. Try a variety of stretches to keep your shoulders, pectoral muscles, and upper back relaxed and free. When you do your gentle breathing meditation, place your hand over your heart chakra. If you are with someone else, one of you can lie down while the other sits and places his or hand over the first person's heart chakra. You can do this on the chest or upper back. Then both of you can do your gentle breathing meditation.

PRACTICAL EXERCISES

1. Practice sitting and standing with a relaxed but upright back, chin tucked in slightly, the top of your head pushed up gently, and your shoulders slightly pulled back. Experiment with this posture until you feel that your heart center is comfortably open.
2. Practice your gentle breathing meditation, initiating each in and out breath, with one hand over your heart.
3. Practice working with a friend. One person lies flat; the other places his or her hand on the first person's chest or upper back. Both people then do the gentle breathing meditation.
4. Try bringing yourself gently to an orgasm while making love, and being aware of how your energy moves and mixes with that of your lover.

SUMMARY

1. The heart, center of the chest, is where we often feel love and emotions.
2. Simply opening our hearts allows energy to flow freely between body and mind. This can be healing in itself.
3. Listening to our hearts develops our intuition.
4. In traditional Indian thinking, we have seven main chakras, or energy centers.
5. The heart chakra is the central chakra; when open it allows energy to flow freely between the lower three chakras and the upper three.
6. We can get a feel for our chakras and the way they open through making love.
7. By opening our hearts and feeling our souls, we can find our own truths and use them to help make decisions and choices in life.
8. When our heart chakras open we can feel universal love.
9. Posture, gentle breathing meditation, and healing help open this chakra.

CHAPTER SIXTEEN
Accepting Emotions

Some people think macrobiotics means permanently eating a restricted diet, but I think that misses the point. Macrobiotics literally means living life to its fullest, so as long as the majority of my diet is fresh food and whole grains, I eat as much chocolate and pizza as I like.

Finding an optimal balance extends to other aspects of life as well. It's impossible to enjoy "the big life" if you don't get enough sleep, or have a backlog of jobs you never finish.

When I take care of my own needs in this way, I have more time and energy to appreciate what I've been given. Then I notice ways I can give, and that's when life becomes truly fulfilling.

—JAN MOSBACHER, founder of Bowden House Community

Emotions tend to come and go like clouds in the sky. There are numerous possible influences on our emotional states. Events, people, memories, food, environment, weather, seasons, and lunar cycles can all affect our moods. Associations may trigger some emotions, as sometimes we get into a habit of responding in a certain way to a particular event. For me, it can be problems with my computer. As soon something starts to go wrong, I assume the worst and feel quite frustrated and, later, feel a persistent doom and gloom or depression.

In a healing session, we might find emotional energy coming up to the surface that brings out strong emotions with it. This can lead to crying, sadness, and painful memories. With practice, we can learn how to experience more of the emotions we feel happy with—as our emotions come from within and, ultimately, we create them ourselves—but I suspect that for most people, most of the time, it feels as though the emotions find us.

When we use our macrobiotic ideals of not making assumptions, giving things meanings, or being dualistic in our thinking, we would then want to just accept the emotion rather than judge it. Many people have written about the dangers of suppressing emotions and burying them deep inside our bodies. This is most likely to happen when we cannot accept an emotion. We may feel that it would be wrong to experience anger, rage, sadness, tears, or grief—so we suppress them. We may find that we have learned through experience to continually suppress certain emotions without even knowing it. I remember suppressing many childhood emotions at school; this has resulted in me putting on a certain emotional face with friends and finding it harder to let go and cry when I feel like it.

Similarly, we might find it uncomfortable to be around someone who is letting his or her emotions come to the surface. Social etiquette has encouraged us to be emotionally restrained and to see certain emotions has being undesirable.

I would suggest that the first step to emotional healing is to accept our emotions just as they are and to express them freely. Just feel them and appreciate them in the knowledge that they will pass. This prevents you from suppressing ongoing emotions and allows you to let some of the old emotional energy leave your body.

Anything that helps move our energies and blood will, in theory, assist us in allowing our emotions to move on. Stretching and exercise can both introduce the movement we need to make it easier to let go of unwanted emotions. Being around other people can sometimes have a similar effect.

STRETCHING

Try ten or twenty minutes of long, slow stretches each day. This will help keep your physical body more flexible and allow your blood to flow more easily. Each shape you adopt in your stretch will also put your energetic body into a new shape, and make it easier to feel different emotions and let go of certain emotions. Be aware of your emotions during each stretch.

Stretch each area of your body, including your neck, shoulders, arms, back, chest, abdomen, groin, and legs. You can stretch while standing, sitting, kneeling, or lying on the floor. Hanging off a bar is a good way to stretch the upper body. Make each stretch slow and gentle. Hold each stretch for about ten seconds. Avoid any sudden movements, and make sure you are stable and secure.

EXERCISE

See if you can find an enjoyable exercise routine that elevates your heartbeat and breathing rate but isn't so vigorous that you can't hold a conversation with someone while doing it. This might include fast walking, swimming, aerobics, or playing sports. The idea is to get your blood flowing more quickly, to see if this helps you bring old, buried emotions up to the surface and accept them. This should help you release emotional energy more easily.

If you can exercise outside in a park, field, or woods, you may find it easier to connect with the surrounding energy and use this to accept emotions. Swimming in the sea or fresh water can help us release emotions. When in the water, some of the free electrons buzzing around our bodies find their way into the water, literally giving away some of our energy. Again, compare your emotions before and after exercising to see what changes you experience.

HEALING

Working with another person can help bring emotions to the surface. The simplest way to do this is for one person to lie down and for the other person to sit comfortably and place one hand over the heart chakra, either on the chest or upper back. Then, both people can go into the gentle breathing meditation while the person sitting places his or her free hands wherever feels appropriate: this could be the lower back, abdomen, forehead, shoulders, top of the head, back of the head, hands, or knees.

After a while, your hands may feel hot as energy passes between you. If both of you can keep coming back to your meditation and find that state of universal love, all kinds of emotions can float up to the surface; in my experience, in this state they are easier to accept and release.

TALKING

Talking with people can also help accept and release emotions. When doing this, it's important to find someone who's good at listening and able to gently probe you to explore further. Someone who adds in his or her own opinions and tries to persuade you to see things his or her way can make the situation worse.

Depending how they have been trained, even professional therapists sometimes have a conceptual agenda. For example, some might see all your emotions as relating to unresolved childhood issues, another might look to your relationships with your parents, and yet another might see your way of thinking as most important. Each of these frameworks add another conceptual layer, and risk making it harder for us to connect with our souls.

PRACTICAL EXERCISES

1. Practice just feeling and accepting emotions without passing any kind of judgment. Try to explore solely the feeling of that emotion.
2. Be prepared to let buried emotions come up to the surface as you become more aware of them.
3. Practice not letting social pressure encourage you to suppress emotions.
4. Talk about your emotional feelings to someone who is good at just listening.
5. Stretch for ten minutes a day to help you feel different emotions and feel different about your emotions.
6. Regular exercise is helpful for stirring up our energetic bodies and buried emotions.
7. Try a healing session to encourage deep, buried emotions to come up to the surface and be released.

SUMMARY

1. Emotions come and go.
2. Though we may be influenced by various outside forces, we ultimately choose our own emotions.
3. By accepting all of our emotions, we reduce the risk of suppressing them and make it easier to release them.

4. We may have learned to suppress and bury our emotions to conform to social conventions.

5. Stretching can pull our emotional energy fields into different shapes and help us release emotions.

6. Stretching also opens up our muscles, making it easier to release emotions.

7. Exercise stirs up the blood and also helps stir up old, stagnant emotions.

8. Talking to a good listener can be therapeutic in itself.

9. Sharing healing sessions with someone can help bring deep, buried emotions up to the surface in a way that makes it easier to release them.

CHAPTER SEVENTEEN
Emotions and Natural Influences

I am grateful each and every day that I had opportunity to have macrobiotics in my life. Not only because of food that makes my family, and
children strong and healthy but because it reminds me about joy in life
that we have to find in simple things. After twenty-five years I am still
amazed with the fact that one cup of simple tea with umeboshi can completely change my condition. And sharing that experience during lectures
and cooking classes brought special treasure in my life. Anyone who
needs or seeks inspiration for taking responsibility of his or her own life
can find it in Macrobiotic philosophy.

—JADRANKA BOBAN PEJIĆ, author, teacher,
and cofounder of Makronova Institute, Zagreb, Croatia

Many cultures have observed the world we know and tried to work out how it
affects us. What effect do the natural forces around us have on our emotions?
Chinese philosophy and medicine has explored the ways we connect to the
world and tried to describe it in terms of yin and yang as well as the five elements. We will explore these later, in the Part Five.

The dilemma that we have is that while different factors have been demonstrated to influence our emotions, and most of us can probably relate to feeling different depending on something like the weather, it would be
disempowering to assume that our emotions are controlled by outside forces.
In fact, we also know through experience that we do control our emotions, and
we can do that regardless of how exterior influences change the way we feel.
For me, the point is that we can make it easier to feel a certain way if we're aware
of the natural forces around us. Just as it might be harder to feel tranquil after
a strong cup of coffee and a slice of sugary cake, we might find a busy shopping mall on the day of the full moon a slightly harder place to meditate.

The key concept here is awareness. I'm proposing that you develop an awareness of whether your emotions are consistently influenced by exterior forces and, if so, how you respond. Ultimately, it would help to be aware of how you can use these forces to encourage the emotions you want to cultivate.

SUN

The sun provides us with light, warmth, and solar radiation. It's the source of our energy, and our exposure to the sun can influence our moods. Some people will go to great lengths to seek out sunshine to lift their mood and escape the winter. Sunshine helps us make vitamin D, and a lack of sun can, for some, lead to abnormal serotonin and melatonin levels contributing to depression.

The sun is the heart of our solar system, and being able to see and feel it can help us feel warm and connected. In Chinese philosophy, the sun radiates fire chi that helps bring our emotions to the surface.

WEATHER

Perhaps the biggest changes to our emotions come from electrical storms: the strong negative charge at the bottom of clouds and the opposite charge of the ground create strong currents of energy and an excitement we can feel in the atmosphere. Walking outside on a windy day can blow away some of the energy that surrounds us. This can feel mentally and emotionally refreshing, almost as though the wind blows our some of our outer energy and emotions away. Sometimes soft rain and low clouds can feel gently soothing. Walking outside and getting wet effectively grounds us, letting us get rid of free electrons and free radicals. Clouds and wind create a moving sky that brings change and variety. This can sometimes subtly help us feel more open to change.

TIMES OF DAY

We can react in different ways to different times of day. Some of us will thrive in the morning; others may do their best work at night. It's interesting to be aware of how you feel in the morning, in the afternoon, in the evening, and at night. I find that being out in nature at different times of day amplifies whatever I might usually feel at that time.

You could try going out into nature as the sun rises, at midday, during the afternoon, at sunset, and during the night. Being out in nature at night can be an interesting emotional experience. On a clear night, we can see our universe above while all around is quiet. For me, this creates an interesting mixture of being highly aware of myself while also being aware of my place in the cosmos. My own problems take on a new perspective when compared to the size of our universe.

SEASONS

Statistically, the seasons have an effect on our behavior. We're more likely to start a new diet or do something to improve our health at the beginning of spring. In many cultures, educational programs start in the autumn. We tend to go out more in the summer and stay in more and sleep more in the winter. The seasons help us move through different emotional phases and encourage us to accept different emotional energies.

We already have a lifetime's experience of living through the seasons; we can remember how we felt at different times of year to find out how we respond to each season. This will be useful when we study the five elements.

Although we might have our preferences for a particular season, it's by being open to the whole year that we can appreciate the change and opportunity for growth that each season brings. You may find it interesting to reflect on your mood in different seasons and consider what this says about you.

LUNAR CYCLES

The moon's cycle has been shown to have an influence on human behavior. At the time of the full moon, the crime rate increases, car insurance claims go up, and more people seek treatment in hospital emergency rooms. Patients operated on during the full moon are at a slightly higher risk of complications due to bleeding. Some women find their menstrual cycles are influenced by the lunar cycle.

You may find that you feel slightly more stressed, irritable, excitable, expressive, or outgoing during the phase of the full moon, and a little more contemplative, meditative, objective and distant around the time of the new moon. Not everyone experiences this, and some are more affected by it than others.

ENVIRONMENT

Different environments have different atmospheres, and our own emotional energies may react to a change in atmosphere. I find meditating in an empty cathedral helpful for mixing a deep awareness of myself with big ideas. I have found standing on the top of a mountain highly stimulating. For me, sitting under a willow tree by a slow-moving river is particularly calming. Walking though woods helps me think through different ideas. Sailing on the ocean helps me take a very different perspective on life.

You might find that a particular room in your home, a bench in the park, a certain café, or a museum has the kind of atmosphere you respond to. I would suggest that it's helpful to have an awareness of how you feel in different places and be able to use your experience to find a place to go when you want to make it a little easier to experience certain emotions.

CLOTHING

The clothes we wear are inside our fields of energy. So, in theory, their colors, shapes, and the fabrics they are made from can subtly influence our moods. You may have had the experience of going home and changing your clothes and feeling different. Sometimes getting dressed up for a special event can in itself change your mood.

You may find it easiest to be aware of the effects of clothing on your mood when changing from extremes: for example, from formal work clothes to loose, relaxing clothes; from bright colors to pale shades; from wool to cotton to synthetics; from lots of jewelry to none at all. It's also interesting to observe how people relate to you when you wear different types of clothing.

With experience, you could choose certain clothes to subtly help you feel the emotions you are looking for. Perhaps a loose, cream-colored outfit helps you meditate, or a tight purple top feels more exciting.

ELECTROMAGNETIC FIELDS

Other factors that might subtly affect our moods are electromagnetic fields (EMFs), electrical radiation, and radio waves. This is a growing issue as our exposure to these items increases. Essentially, all of these fields introduce extra free electrons to our bodies, which can affect the quality of the cells they enter. In the process, we may feel different.

For example, after you've spent a day in an office, shopping mall, or hospital, compare how you feel to your mood after spending a day in the countryside, at a beach, or in a park. You might also find that making long calls on a cell phone changes the way you feel.

The best way to reduce your exposure to EMFs and electrical radiation is to keep away from electrical appliances, including computers, televisions, stereos, lights, electric cooking appliances, electric heaters, fax machines, copiers, and electrical outlets that are in use. You often only need to be one yard or meter away from an appliance to be outside its field. This is most important for your sleeping space. Try to ensure that there's no electrical equipment near your head and, to a lesser extent, your body when you lie in your bed. See if you can move equipment to at least a yard or meter away. You can apply the same principle to any place you sit for a long time.

When using a cell phone, hold the phone away from you while it's connecting and starting the call, as this is when it sends out the strongest signal. Try to keep your calls short. More frequent short calls may be less damaging than one or two very long calls. Send text messages as much as possible instead of making calls. Be careful about moving to a home close to a cell phone tower. Try not to stand close to a microwave oven when it is use. Also, clothing made from synthetic fibers can carry a charge of static electricity, adding to the electrical fields within and around you.

It may be that having lots of plants in your home helps reduce your exposure to EMFs. Grounding yourself by taking baths or showers, walking barefoot, or swimming can help drain away some of the extra electrons your body picks up.

Most important, try not to get attached to any possible connection between your emotions and the surrounding energy. Remember, you ultimately have the power to create your own emotions; to feel that you are somehow under the control of the energy around you would disempower you from feeling that sense of control over your emotions.

PRACTICAL EXERCISES

1. Be aware of how you feel on a sunny day compared to a cloudy day.
2. Make a note in your diary of the weather and your emotions to see if they are connected.
3. Be aware of your energy levels and emotions at different times of the day note whether there's a consistent pattern.
4. Write out how you feel in each season.
5. Get a calendar with the full and new moon indicated. Note any changes in your mood between the phases. Women might find it interesting to note whether their menstrual cycle is at the time of the full or new moon.
6. Whenever you go to a public building, note your emotions along with a brief description of the type of building you are in. After a few months, review your notes to see if there is any connection between your environment and mood.
7. Try wearing dramatically different styles of clothing and be aware of any changes in your emotions. Make notes in your diary so you can see which clothes help you feel certain emotions.
8. Compare being in an artificial environment with plenty of EMFs, electrical radiation, and radio waves to being in a natural environment. Try being in a shopping mall, hospital, or office; and then spend a similar amount of time out in nature.
9. Move any electrical equipment or wires so they are at least one yard or meter away from your bed and anywhere else you spend a lot of time.

10. Keep your cell phone away from your head while it's connecting to make a call. Text instead of making calls. Keep calls as short as possible.

11. Connect your body to the earth regularly by walking barefoot on the ground, taking baths and showers, swimming, or doing an activity that brings you into direct contact with the earth, such as gardening.

12. Experiment with finding out how much you can choose your own emotions in any situation.

SUMMARY

1. Many cultures have explored the ways we are connected to our universe.

2. These connections are influences and do not prevent us from taking control of our own emotions.

3. External influences could include the sun, weather, time of day, seasons, lunar cycles, environment, clothing, EMFs, other people, and food.

4. By creating an awareness of how each of these affects us, we can start to think about how we're connected to the world around us and how we can use our experience to help create the emotions we want to cultivate.

5. At the same, time we ultimately have the ability to choose our own emotional state and override external influences.

CHAPTER EIGHTEEN

Society, Friends, Family, and Children

I started practicing macrobiotics in the 1980s and was amazed by the sense of well-being and increased energy that I quickly experienced. The foods and dishes taste absolutely delicious and are packed with nutrition and vitality. I have raised seven children on organic, living foods, and can happily say I am still alive to tell the tale! My children are strong, intelligent, and self-motivated. They rarely get sick and, if they do, they recover quickly. Macrobiotic foods provide a strong foundation for mental, emotional, and physical health. When we take responsibility for our well-being, we also feel empowered and in control of our lives. Eating grains, beans, and vegetables gives us a direct link to the energy of the earth, one that helps us to feel stable, secure, and connected. Macrobiotics begins in the home, starting with the self and then broadening out to our children, our friends, and our community. It really is a marvelous way to enjoy and relish life.

—MELANIE BROWN WAXMAN, macrobiotic teacher, counselor, and cook, and author of *The Cooklets*, *Bless the Baby*, *Yummy Yummy in My Tummy*, and *Eat Me Now!*

Archeologists and anthropologists speculate that humans have been able to survive only by working together. It appears that primitive man did not have the natural ability to hunt by himself and, if anything, spent more time avoiding being eaten by other creatures than finding food. Because our young take so long to grow and develop to a point where they can take care of themselves, mothers and children would have been particularly vulnerable to attack. Given this, our greatest chance of survival was to form communities and share the role of looking after the young and going out to collect food.

It seems that our earliest diets revolved around collecting vegetables, roots, and fruits before moving on to harvesting grains, beans, nuts, and seeds. Meat and fish were harder to come by until we invented hunting weapons. Food collection naturally works well when performed in teams, and by the time we started to use agriculture, a simple society was well established.

It's likely that being able to form and work in a team is wired into our DNA for our survival. You might find that many of your basic character traits are there to help you integrate into society. Watching children develop, it becomes clear how many social skills are already in place, ready to come out in the playground. Your smile, desire to help, ability to make people laugh, leadership qualities, need to be valued, desire to be useful, ability to make friends, and so on may all be there to help you be part of a community that at one time would have been essential for the survival of yourself and your babies. In turn, our children would have been our pension and, once grown, essential to help in times of ill health and old age.

Our desire to communicate may be born out of a basic instinct to warn each other of danger and pass on our successes so that our whole community might prosper. In my humble opinion, suppressing these natural instincts is unhealthy. By joining in, being a part of the conversation, playing together, sharing in the fun, and expressing ourselves, we can productively and creatively use and nourish some of our most primal energies.

Interestingly, scientists claim that our cells contain a number of organelles (for example, mitochondria) that used to be bacteria with individual lives; now, they have evolved to work as a community inside every human cell. Mitochondria will even commit suicide for the well-being and health of the whole body. When the mitochondria become selfish and do not give in to the common good, cells risk becoming cancerous. So it may be that our whole bodies are based on separate living entities all trying to work together as a community. To explore this topic further, I recommend *Power, Sex, Suicide: Mitochondria and the Meaning of Life* by Nick Lane.

Today it's no longer strictly necessary for us to be a part of a community; it's possible to live on our own, work individually, and grow old without a family. However, I suggest that by being part of a community we nourish our deepest self. Being part of a society for the sake of it does have challenges of its own— it can be a great source of stress. But I would propose that enjoying being part of a community and being a valued member is in itself healing, and through being with people we can find the feedback and support that keeps us on our healing journey.

A traditional part of being social is communal eating, whether at a dinner party, in a restaurant, or while on vacation. If you feel secure in your macrobiotic eating, there's no reason not to enjoy different forms of social eating—and ultimately, in the broadest sense of healing, it may be healthier to do so.

BEING IN SERVICE

One of the ways we become part of a community is by being in service: making ourselves available to others and, in a way, surrendering our individual needs to the needs of the group. In one way, this act has appeared to have been taken over by governments and charities; however, I think we all have much to gain by being able to offer ourselves to a group of people directly without expecting anything in return, rather than simply handing over money.

Melanie Brown Waxman, my life partner Dragana, and I run a macrobiotics discussion group set up by our friend Bruce Paine and, although it can be time-consuming, it has also been extremely rewarding emotionally. Through our group we've met hundreds of people around the globe and created an environment where we can share our experiences and support each other without any expectations. Many other teachers have joined in, including many of those quoted in this book. All have been happy to be of service to those joining the macrobiotic community.

I recommend finding ways that you can enjoy being of service to people. Try simply being there for someone else: being supportive, kind, and gentle—in essence, just giving of yourself. Practical examples would include volunteering to help look after children, doing chores or other needed tasks for the elderly, initiating community projects, helping out at a charity, or simply being a good neighbor and making that little extra effort to see if people need help. You could also put yourself in service to a group of people trying to improve our environment, taking on a political campaign, or bringing about constructive social change in another way.

ISOLATION

One of the big problems in the practice of macrobiotics is isolation. Sometimes people feel like they have taken on a new life and become a different person after starting to eat macrobiotically. They often feel a great desire to share this experience, and if others aren't interested, it can be a lonely existence.

My observation is that people in this situation also risk losing the natural feedback system of listening to other people. Those close to us who do not understand the macrobiotic path we have chosen can feel threatened and seem defensive or negative. The result can be that we feel defensive and as if we constantly have to explain ourselves; it can sometimes result in a kind of contracted emotional energy that I would suggest is not healthy. As a result, we may choose to isolate ourselves in order to avoid having to explain our different behavior. My advice would be to enjoy your practice of macrobiotics, and simply communicate about it in terms of your feelings. No one can argue with a statement like, "Since eating this way, I just feel a lot better."

If you want to start practicing macrobiotics, I recommend using the Internet to seek out macrobiotic centers, people, teachers, and activities near you. If you join an Internet discussion group, you can ask questions and hopefully find someone near to you. You can organize potluck dinners, picnics, or simply gatherings with other people who also enjoy macrobiotics.

Ultimately, it will help to build a network of people you can trust to tell you when you might be looking too thin, seeming uptight, becoming obsessive about food, taking it all too seriously, or being too strict with yourself. Listen to comments and without being defensive, and try to use them to reflect on your own state.

TRIBES

It's a natural human tendency to want to join a tribe. If we meet a group of people doing something similar to what we're doing, we often feel compelled to join them—a bit like joining a gang at school. In 1984 I moved to Philadelphia to live with Melanie, and I definitely became part of the macrobiotic tribe. Later,

I returned to London to run the East West Centre; I continued living in the macrobiotic tribe and lost contact with my previous friends.

For me, being part of the macrobiotic tribe was exhilarating, stimulating, and exciting. We invited many macrobiotic teachers to London, and it was part of my job to look after them; many became lasting friends. The other side to this was that being surrounded by people who had similar beliefs to mine, there was no one in my life to effectively challenge me. In addition, the tribe tended to become more isolated from the rest of society while we perpetuated our belief systems by continually supporting each other.

It was only later, when I temporarily left my macrobiotic tribe and reconnected with some of my old friends and family, that I could take a different perspective. By stepping out of the tribe I was able examine and analyze many of my macrobiotic beliefs. Out of this, I was better able to discover my own interpretation of macrobiotics and live it myself rather than be influenced by other people's beliefs. When I rejoined the macrobiotic tribe, I found many of my macrobiotic friends had been on a similar journey.

In a way, tribes and isolation are a complementary pair. Too much of one can require a dose of the other. If I were starting my macrobiotics practice over again with what I have learned, I'd make a bigger effort to not only enjoy making friends within the macrobiotic community but also to maintain other friendships so I could keep a better perspective on life. I would seek out those who could challenge me and help me maintain an open and big view. I think it's a natural inclination to want to dig deeper and deeper into a subject, and sometimes this can result in us becoming buried in it. Sometimes we need a friend to come along and pull us out of the hole so we can see the big picture again.

FRIENDS

One of the social challenges some people have faced is that when eating macrobiotically and having a wonderful experience, there arises a desire for everyone else to have the same experience. As we discussed earlier, it's natural to want to tell everyone about our success.

Humans tend to have something of a herd mentality, and we feel safe if we are all eating similar foods, sharing similar values and having similar attitudes toward life. If one of our herd then decides to take on a new diet and a new outlook on life, and even questions some of our accepted ideas on health, it can be threatening to the rest of the group. Your friends and family might feel uncomfortable with your starting a macrobiotic lifestyle. When one of Dragana's school friends became vegetarian, her mother took her to a psychiatrist.

Upsetting those around you doesn't help your journey, and I would advise anyone starting a macrobiotics practice to share your own experience of macrobiotics while being considerate of other people's feelings. Avoid trying to convert anyone and, in particular, don't criticize someone else's diet or way of life; this will lead only to the other person becoming defensive and finding ways to attack you. I would suggest that you feel comfortable and content in what you do, resist imposing yourself on others, and help those who ask.

FAMILY AND CHILDREN

If you're the only member of your family eating macrobiotically and you're worried about how your partner and children will respond, remind yourself that we are each on our own journey through life. I certainly grew up with what would in macrobiotic terms be considered an unhealthy diet, and, although I did experience some minor health issues, I'm still alive and feeling healthy now. This is true for most people in the macrobiotic community.

It helps to keep food in perspective and remember that good relationships with our immediate family might be more important to our health than whether or not those around us eat a helping of brown rice. If you can encourage your children to eat plenty of vegetables and some fruit every day, you will already have taken a giant step forward in terms of healthy eating. Any other macrobiotic foods are just a bonus. It has been my observation that children who have been brought up on a restrictive version of the macrobiotic diet have run into more problems than those who've been given more freedom and explored a wider interpretation.

I think it's helpful to introduce your children to as wide and varied a diet as possible. It's through experiencing many different foods that children can begin to have their own awareness of food, which will lead to them developing their own intuition. Raising children on a strict macrobiotic diet denies them the benefits of exploring a wide variety of foods and, ultimately, of finding which foods are best for them. Instead, they may just eat a diet that works for you and suffer as a result.

Dragana and I tried to encourage our children to at least try different foods each time they were served. A common problem is that if a child tries a food once and doesn't like it, he or she assumes that food will never taste good. The child will make the claim, "I don't like pumpkin," or radishes, or whatever the food is. In reality, the child can only say that he or she didn't like the food prepared in the way it was at that particular meal. The next day, the ingredients might taste different or be cooked differently, and the child's own taste might have changed according to his or her mood.

I would recommend finding a way to encourage your children to at least try one bite, even if they have eaten similar food before and not liked it. Children and adults are very good at acquiring the taste for foods. Growing up I didn't like the taste of coffee, beer, wine, and Stilton cheese, among other things, but over time I acquired a taste for them and even came to like them too much for a while. Similarly, I did not like miso soup, natto, or adzuki beans when I first tried them, but with a little effort I acquired the taste for them; they have become favorites. The same can happen with children if we can find a positive way to encourage them to at least try a small amount on a regular basis.

When we restrict a food, we tend to make it more desirable. Having food in the house and then telling a child that he or she can have it only as a treat will make that food highly desirable. My suggestion is to try having a wide variety of generally healthy foods in your home and letting your children feel free to eat them. The only eating rule we had was that the children could eat any snacks as long as they could still eat their meals.

When we went out, we would let the children eat anything they wanted. They would order ice cream, sugary desserts, all kinds of pizza, and so on.

When they were young, we were still in a phase of feeling cautious over meat; even though I still have not tried any myself, I felt comfortable with my children trying it. Personally, I was aware that I didn't want to impose my ideas on them. At the same time, as their parent I wanted to create an environment where they felt happy to eat a generally healthy diet by choice.

SOCIAL EATING

There's something interesting about spending time with other people and eating the same food together. When a group of people eat the same food, they have something in common. Many societies have rituals and celebrations that often include eating together. I suspect there's something special about the way our emotional energy mixes when we share food. I therefore encourage anyone practicing macrobiotics to make an effort to eat with your family, and join in on social occasions even if it means compromising your usual food choices. As long as we have built up a relationship with the healthy foods we want to eat, the occasional diversion for the sake of social unity is unlikely to harm us.

Restaurants and Holidays

Similarly, eating out from time to time is perfectly compatible with living macrobiotically. In fact, I would suggest that it's healthier to eat out with friends sometimes than to feel confined to your own kitchen, even if it means eating foods you would not normally have. In addition, we live in a time when it's easier than ever to eat out healthily. I have found that I can eat at Japanese, Italian, Indian, Thai, Chinese, French, Moroccan, Swiss, and Greek restaurants and find plenty of dishes that feel healthy to me.

You could apply the same idea to holidays. As a family, we enjoy traveling, experiencing different cultures, and enjoying local foods. For me, it's a great way to try new foods and feel their effects. Through our travels we have adopted many new dishes. I think it's healthy to go through a period of experiencing different foods and have a break from the usual dietary routine. I've also noticed that when we come home I have a greater enthusiasm to get back to my familiar soups, whole grains, and vegetable dishes.

COMPARISONS AND COMPETITION

One of the ways we can create difficulties in being around other people is when we make comparisons. By comparing ourselves to others we risk distracting ourselves from our true purpose in life; we invite false reasons to gloat or feel inferior. It's very easy to sucked into the games we play in social situations. Who's got the biggest house, fastest car, best husband? Humans are prone to trying to discover what the rules are and then competing. Perhaps it's wired into us from birth; I've noticed children left on their own will soon invent a game and make up rules.

Check out whether you're living your life and taking the journey you want, or whether you've become caught up in a game and your heart isn't really in it. How much do looks, wealth, achievements, holidays, or material things really mean to you? You might find that you even transfer your desire to compare and compete to your children's successes. Does your son or daughter winning a competition, award, or prize mean more to you than it does to them?

Ideally we would each live the life that feels right to us and stay true to ourselves regardless of what other people are doing. See if you can catch yourself making comparisons, and whether you can relax and just accept yourself as you are instead.

EGO

It can be quite a challenge to interact with other people without our egos getting in the way. It's very easy to want to impress, be liked, command respect, or win friends. In pursuit of this, we may present ourselves in ways that are not entirely honest. The problem is that we create a mask that prevents us from really connecting with another person.

I would highly recommend trying to be with someone without feeling the need to please, make an impression, or put on an act. You might find this easier if you practice the breathing meditation, get into your heart, and take this feeling into your interactions with other people.

With practice you may find you can simply listen to your friend and respond from your heart. When you do this you will bypass your ego and be your true self. The interactions that occur on this level can add a new dimension to your friendships.

FEELING LOVE

When two people are feeling their heart energy, a kind of magnetic attraction occurs. In this state, you might experience a pleasant feeling of love. You can try this out by practicing your gentle breathing meditation with another person using an exercise I once learned with a qi gong master and then more recently at an esoteric healing course. Once you both feel able to focus solely on your breathing for about twenty or thirty seconds at a time, you can try this exercise.

Stand facing each other, about two feet or sixty centimeters apart. Close your eyes just to get used to the sensation. Both of you then go into your breathing meditation, and try to focus on the energy of your chest and your heart chakra. As you do this, be aware of your balance. You may find that you both feel an attraction and that your weight moves forward onto your toes. Sometimes you'll experience strong pulls toward each other.

Try again standing back to back: close your eyes, and, when you are in your heart meditation, see whether you both feel like you are falling backwards toward each other.

Whenever you are in a social situation that feels difficult, try going into your gentle breathing meditation; you may find that the energy of your interaction quickly changes. If you can connect with another person with your soul and love, it is harder for someone to want to harm you.

LAUGHTER

A popular claim is that laughter is the best medicine. I feel that laughter is an instant way to relieve stress—it's a lot quicker and less expensive than having a massage! When we're with friends, we have great opportunities to joke, be playful, and have fun. We can share the energy of laughter, which is quite infectious; I notice this when I am around someone who laughs a lot. I also find it healthy to be able to laugh at myself—and all we do in the field of macrobiotics. On that note, I'd like to make a special thanks to all the comedians who have made me laugh so much, especially two in our own small community, Verne Varona and Jessica Porter, who also contributed to this book.

PRACTICAL EXERCISES

1. Do something that puts you into a situation where you are of service to others.
2. Use the Internet to see if there are macrobiotic activities, people, and community near you.
3. Make a point of being open to hearing your friends' and family members' comments about you.
4. Make a list of ways it might upset your family when you starting to eat macrobiotically, and use this to be understanding of them.
5. See if you can get your children to try some vegetables and a piece of fruit every day.
6. Try keeping a wide range of healthy foods and snacks in your home for your children.
7. Invite friends around for a tasty macrobiotic meal.
8. Make a point of eating out and finding something you feel is healthy on the menu.
9. Make a list of the ways you compare yourself to other people. Reflect on the effect this has on you.
10. Make a list of ways you compete with other people, and note the effect this has on your life.
11. Make a list of ways you try to impress other people, and try to be aware of when you're doing it.
12. Practice the exercise of standing close to different people while in your gentle breathing meditation, and be aware of the way you feel.

SUMMARY

1. For our own and our children's survival, we have a long history of living together and working in teams.

2. The need to live together has meant we have evolved complex social skills that may be inherent in us from birth.

3. Our desire to communicate may come from primitive urges to protect and improve a community.

4. We can nurture our primal social instincts by being in service of other people.

5. One of the challenges of practicing macrobiotics is that we can feel isolated and, through this, lose an important feedback system.

6. We have the opportunity, through the Internet, to find macrobiotic activities, meet people eating macrobiotically, and join Internet discussion groups.

7. You may want to join a macrobiotic tribe, and in doing so you may lose contact with older friends and end up inside a macrobiotic bubble, apart from the rest of society.

8. When you feel good, you may want to tell everyone about macrobiotics; this can produce a negative reaction if other people are already feeling threatened or insecure about your change of lifestyle. However, people are less likely to feel upset if you just communicate the way you feel eating your new foods.

9. Attacking other people's diets tends to make them defensive and want to attack your diet.

10. It's important to keep a sense of perspective and accept that loved ones eating foods you do not consider healthy may still enjoy excellent health.

11. Encouraging your children to eat some vegetables and a piece of fruit every day will already be a big step forward, and any other healthy changes will be a bonus.

12. Try to get your children to keep trying foods, even if they did not like a certain food previously. Their relationship to a food can change depending on how it is prepared.

13. If we restrict others or ourselves from a certain food, the risk is that it becomes more desirable.

14. One option is to keep healthy foods at home and let children eat whatever they like when out.

15. It's healthy to go out and eat with friends.

16. Going on holiday is a good opportunity to try different dishes.

17. Comparing ourselves to others can create problems.

18. Following our desires to compete can lead us away from our true purposes in life.

19. Our egos often get in the way of having real interactions with people, as we try to create a certain impression.

20. Talking from our hearts can create stronger and closer connections.

21. Two people standing close to each other with their eyes closed will feel a physical attraction to each other when meditating and feeling love in their hearts.

CHAPTER NINETEEN
Emotional Energy

When I began practicing macrobiotics forty years ago, I was inspired by the philosophy and its promise of freedom. The foods, then, were a practical discipline for developing my understanding of life. Thanks to the unique philosophy of yin and yang, I became more independent in my thinking and judgment. The freedom has been from fears and popular opinions. Since I have devoted my life to teaching and counseling many thousands of people, including using acupuncture, I have gained many insights into human nature and needs, including my own. So my dietary practices have evolved from an ultra-strict and limited diet to one that is much more flexible and intuitive. I remain very grateful to macrobiotics for offering a truly large view of life, and remain inspired to refine and develop myself ever further.

—MICHAEL ROSSOFF, LAc, macrobiotic teacher and counselor

In the theory of the energy body, our energies become disturbed when we experience an upsetting event. Sometimes our bodies remember this and maintain an association with similar experiences and disturbances. For example, someone might almost fall out of a window and experience a great disturbance in his or her energetic body, along with upsetting emotions. Then every time he or she goes near a window again, he or she might experience the same disturbances and feel upset, even though there is no risk of falling out of the window.

Similar things can happen with food. We might build up an association with a food and, because of this, find it very hard to break whatever pattern we have of relating to the food. For example, I might get into the habit of relaxing after my evening meal and eating some chocolate. After a while, I may find that I have built up strong associations between feeling relaxed and content after my meal and the taste of chocolate. If I can break the association, I will then be in a better position to choose not to eat the chocolate.

In this chapter we will explore ways to break those connections so we can feel freer to make the choices we want in life.

ASSOCIATIONS

All through life we form associations with different things. Many of these may have been formed in childhood and go back to our relationships with our parents. Sometimes these associations can come to work against us. We may associate receiving gifts as a child with being loved, for example, and then find that in adulthood we need someone to give us presents to feel loved.

We may have very strong emotional associations with lots of different foods. These can come about through having had treats as a child, eating certain snacks while we relax, or having some special treat when eating out. We may also have used these associations to help overcome energetic and emotional disturbances. For example, when we're feeling stressed, we might reach for a box of cookies because we've already built up an association between eating cookies and feeling relaxed. Stress causes an emotional upset and cookies, with their calming association, would be the remedy we use to feel better again.

One way to work with this is to build up new associations with foods you would prefer to be eating. To do this, you could make a point of listening to your favorite music, watching a comedy, or reading a romantic book while eating a certain food so that you come to associate these emotions with it. Eventually, you will turn to your new food when craving those happy emotions.

It would also make sense to look at what associations are linked to the stress in the first place, and explore whether there's a pattern that could be broken. Sometimes the cause of stress is irrational. Someone else eating in a certain way, dressing in particular fashion, or having a certain attitude toward life can bring up unpleasant, stressful associations.

ACUPRESSURE POINTS

One of the ways we can calm our energetic bodies is through the use of acupressure points. These are points on the skin where we can help change the flow of energy underneath. This leads to bigger changes in our energies, with the result that we find it easier to experience different emotions.

In acupuncture, the points are precisely located and the energies there are stimulated or calmed by fine metal needles. A simpler way to influence the energy in the body is to tap the bones on which some acupressure points are located. As the tapping vibrates the whole bone, the surrounding energy, including the energy of the acupressure points, will change.

To experience this, you could tap any easy-to-reach bones and see what you feel energetically and emotionally. The most common reaction is to feel calmer and a greater feeling of peace. It may be that as the bones vibrate they allow our energies to move more freely. This has the effect of helping energy that has become constricted, intense, or compressed flow out and disperse. At the same time, spots on your body with a deficiency of energy will benefit from receiving some of the dispersing energy. The end result is that your energy is more evenly distributed and flowing more harmoniously. In a way, when our energies are like this we are more whole, whereas when our energies are bunched up in one place and thin somewhere else we feel fragmented and separate.

We experience free-moving, even energy as contentment, harmoniousness, and wholeness. Through tapping various bones, we can start to feel the kind of emotions we could use when we want to break certain associations. Before we do that, let's become familiar with the easiest bones to reach and the way to tap.

How to Tap

Try tapping with the tips of your fingers. The tapping should be strong enough to vibrate the bones. You can play with making the tapping stronger until you feel an influence; do not tap so strongly that it's painful. It's important to remain relaxed while tapping. If you tap frantically or in a tense way, your energy is unlikely to flow freely. I suggest that you keep your wrist and hand relaxed so that your fingers bounce up and down as you move your arm. Find a comfortable rhythm.

Head

The head is the easiest place to tap, as there are many bones close to the surface. I suggest you start by tapping the top of your head with one or both hands. Then move to the center of your forehead. Next, with two hands, tap each of your temples. From here, you can tap the bones behind your ears and at the back of your head. Then, tap your cheekbones below your eyes. Finally, with one hand, tap between your nose and upper lip, and then on your chin so your whole jaw vibrates.

Chest

The easiest bones on the chest to tap are the collarbones. These run from your shoulders to below the front of your neck. You can also try tapping the ribs just below the collarbones. A powerful point for tapping the chest is in the center, between your nipples.

Back

It's hard to tap your own back, and so you may prefer to leave it out. The best way to reach your lower back is to lean forward and tap with the back of your hands or knuckles.

Hips

Feel your lower back and locate the top of your hips; tap along this ridge to vibrate your pelvic area. In the front, try tapping along the top of your pubic bone.

Legs

The easiest part of the legs to tap is around your knees. There is a powerful acupressure point on the bone below the front of the knee and slightly to the outside. You'll also find useful bones to tap around and above the inside of the ankle.

Hands and Feet

The easiest parts of the hand to tap are the back and side. You can tap along the edge between your little finger and your wrist. The top of the foot is another area with lots of interesting bones to tap. You can explore tapping up from the big toe and along the ridges that run up the top of your foot.

You may find it helps to spend some time tapping different bones, getting used to locating them, and finding the kind of tapping that suits you best. As you try out the tapping, be aware how you feel afterwards. Make a mental note of your emotional state. Use this to discover which bones, when tapped, give you the response you are looking for. You may find after while that you need to tap only a particular bone to feel clam. This may the part of your body where energy gets stuck. Everyone is different, and it's up to you to discover where you need to tap to get the best responses.

EFT

Gary Craig combined the use of acupressure points with therapy to create a technique called Emotional Freedom Techniques (EFT). The idea of EFT is that you relive a traumatic or disturbing event while tapping various bones. By doing this, you can remain calm and keep your energy flowing harmoniously while you re-experience something that would normally disturb you energetically and emotionally. This demonstrates to your subconscious and deeper self that you can be in a challenging situation without feeling upset. It breaks the pattern. The idea is that if you can do this in your imagination, you can then go on to do it in real life.

The process commonly works like this: You start by reliving a situation that is normally upsetting. Be aware of how upsetting it feels. You could even give it a score between one and ten. Then, relive the event while tapping various bones. You could simply tap from head to toe. To keep your mind and subconscious engaged in the event, it is best to describe it out loud. Gary Craig suggests creating a sentence that begins with "Even though" and ends with "I still love and accept myself."

The idea is to be able to relax and love and accept yourself, whatever the situation you are thinking of, and to increase your ability to keep your energy calm. In addition, the "love and accept myself" ending helps reduce the risk of internal conflicts. So, when I feel stressed about, say, the computer not working, I could make up a sentence to describe my feelings. It might go, "Even though I feel stressed that I cannot get an Internet connection, I love and accept myself." I would then say this sentence out loud repeatedly while tapping various bones. As this exercise works with emotions and feelings, I suggest you describe your feelings. For example, I said, "I feel stressed." If my body is able to discover that I can feel calm while I am unable to get an Internet connection then I know deep down that I have this option, as I have already experienced it in my mind.

You could try the same process to break strong emotional associations you have with foods. For example, if you're used to drinking coffee and having a cookie at your morning break and you want to switch to having herbal tea and an apple, you could try tapping while saying, "Even though I feel like coffee and a cookie but would prefer not to have them at my break, I love and accept myself." If you can disconnect the desire for coffee and cookies at a break, you will find it easier to have your herbal tea and apple instead.

You may find that as you are going through the process, saying different sentence feels better. If this happens, change to any new sentence that feels right to you. Sometimes it can be like peeling an onion, and you may find that new issues come up during the process. Feel free to use the same process to try out engaging with an issue while your energetic body remains calm. You may need to repeat the process several times before you can go back to imagining being in the distressing situation without any emotional response.

PRACTICAL EXERCISES

1. Make a list of foods that you eat when you feel upset. Write out any associations you might have built up with these foods.
2. Make a point of creating a happy atmosphere each time you eat food that you would like to be a part of your healthy diet.
3. Practice tapping different bones, and make a note of how you feel before and after.

4. Take an issue you want to change, and create a sentence that begins with "Even though" and ends with "I love and accept myself." Repeat your sentence while tapping various bones.

SUMMARY

1. We have energetic bodies that influence our emotions.
2. We form emotional associations with certain foods and may find ourselves eating those foods just to relive the associated emotions.
3. Once we develop strong emotional associations with foods we no longer want, the associations themselves can make it harder to stop eating them.
4. One way to change this is to consciously make sure that we are in a great mood each time we eat new healthy foods.
5. Acupressure points are places on the body that the Chinese traditionally use to change the energy flow of the energetic body.
6. One way of helping to smooth the flow of our energy is to tap on various bones with the tips of our fingers. This sets up a vibration that encourages energy that is constricted, compressed, or intense to flow into areas where there is a deficiency of energy.
7. You can tap the bones of your head, chest, back, hips, legs, feet, and hands.
8. Emotional Freedom Techniques can help undo emotional associations. EFT is a method of tapping bones to keep your energy calm while reliving an upsetting event. Once you know we can think about an event while remaining calm, you can break the association between the event and being energetically and emotionally disturbed.
9. To relive the event, Gary Craig suggests tapping different bones while repeating a phrase that begins with "Even though" and ends with "I love and accept myself."

CHAPTER TWENTY
Fueling Emotions with Food

With my personal discovery of macrobiotics, I made a life inventory of everything, and I have opened a new chapter in my life. This new inspiration brought me to adopting and developing new skills and initiated the virtue that consequently brought me closer to a sense of dignity. And even further on, while moving in the space of personal imperfections, macrobiotics has supported me in understanding the meaning of self-sufficiency and sustainability. In the critical moments of the past war in Croatia, it motivated me to stand more firmly on the side of peace and nonviolence, as well as to overcome my personal doubts and lack of orientation.

I feel better able to differentiate important things from those less important, to be more responsible, and to be able to take care of my family and myself; this represents the greatest impact of macrobiotic principles on my life. I still feel that macrobiotics gives me enough energy to face the issues that life is about to bring.

—ZLATKO PEJIĆ, health counselor; founder and president of the Society for the Improvement of Quality of Life; cofounder of the Makronova Institute, Zagreb, Croatia; and winner of the 1993 United Nations Earth Day International Award for environmental protection and work toward peace

If we think of food as having its own energy and our emotions as being colored by our energy, then we can explore the idea that the food we eat will in some way influence our energy and therefore also influence our emotions. Michio Kushi illustrates this in lectures by lighting a candle. The wax represents our food; when it combines with the oxygen in the air, energy is created in the form of a flame. Putting something into the wax, like a part of a match, alters the color and size of the flame. Michio would say that in this analogy the flame reflects our emotions.

The idea is that if the energy of the food we eat will subtly influence our emotions, we can then choose foods to help us feel a certain way. To experience this, you may need to eat a certain food consistently and then try another, all while being acutely aware of your emotional state. As the influence of food is mixed up with all the other influences we have explored, it's not always something we're aware of.

ALCOHOL, COFFEE, AND SUGAR

We've already discussed the role of stimulants (for example, alcohol, sugar, coffee) on our minds. These foods can also temporarily open our heart chakras, but in a way that makes it harder to feel and connect to the energy there. The risk is that under the influence of these stimulants we open up our heart centers chaotically and then close them down again. This can ultimately become energetically and emotionally disturbing. We leave ourselves exposed to taking in energies that may not ultimately be what we want while our heart is open and we are not feeling centered.

As we've discussed before, some foods will have a great and clear influence on our emotions, alcohol being the most obvious. Alcohol not only alters our emotional states but leads to feelings of being outside of ourselves. Alcohol presents an opportunity to feel like we're out of our heads, possibly a form of escapism. If you regularly feel like taking on this state, the questions to ask are: Why do you not want to be in yourself? What are you escaping from? I would suggest that to answer these questions, it would help to go back to feeling the soul, feeling that love inside, and feeling whole. In my experience, drinking alcohol makes it harder to feel connected to my soul; when I feel disconnected from my soul, it becomes harder to feel my own truth and use my intuition.

Coffee is another drink that many people know from experience alters our emotions. It seems that coffee can, in some people, raise adrenaline levels and induce a constant state of stress. Too much coffee can put us in a fight-or-flight mode where we feel more reactive, and more likely to snap and feel irritated with people. Too much caffeine can put us in a state where we experience a frenetic, frantic, and even frenzied energy; this makes it difficult to experience the stillness that allows us to connect to our deeper selves and the resources within. The risk is that in this state we make decisions out of a rush of mental energy and ignore our hearts. I would suggest that, to feel your emotions and heart more easily, try not drinking coffee for a few weeks and feel the difference for yourself.

Added sugar has the effect of rapidly increasing blood sugar levels. A gland at the end of the pancreas then starts to secrete insulin, which in turn controls the process of taking sugar out of the blood and into our muscles. When blood sugar rises too quickly, the body overproduces insulin and takes too much sugar out of the blood, leaving us with too little blood sugar. This cycle of rising and falling blood sugar can lead to emotional ups and downs. One cycle can take two to four hours. Once our blood sugar falls to a low, we will experience strong cravings for foods to increase our blood sugar again. This creates a situation where we can feel a rush of sugar-fueled energy and an emotional intensity that is soon followed by feeling flat and distracted by the desire for something sweet. Again, these mood swings take us out of states where we can access our souls and feel our inner beings. In a sense, we feel like we lose control of our emotions and that they are imposed upon us, rather than us being able to choose our emotions.

To help people with diabetes manage their blood sugar with food, there are now tables showing which foods raise blood sugar the quickest and which help maintain steady blood sugar levels. This is discussed fully in Part Five, where we look at the glycemic index and load.

THE ENERGY OF FOODS

In addition to the more obvious influence of stimulants, all foods will have some effect on our emotions. Some foods and dishes will have a greater influence than others. All of this has to be put in perspective, taking into account of the other potential influences and our own ability to create our emotions.

It may be that the living energies of whole foods help us feel different emotions. Most of the macrobiotic foods tend to be whole, and therefore alive up until the time they are cooked or eaten. This means that when we eat these foods, we consume not only their nutrients but also their energies. Whole foods are those that have not been processed, such as vegetables, fruits, dried beans, whole grains, seeds, nuts, and fermented foods. You can read more about these foods in Part Five, when we discuss the living energy in foods.

On a very subtle level, any food can have some influence on our emotions. In theory, there would be a difference between eating a raw carrot and eating an apple; however, the effect would be so small that we would not notice it. You may, however, notice larger differences. For example, eating lots of raw salads, fruit, and vegetables one day and then cooked stews, thick soups, casseroles, and porridge the next day may present enough contrast for you to feel a difference. In my experience, raw foods help me feel lighter and have more of a fresh, "up" feeling. Cooked foods help me feel satisfied, content, and warm.

Another dish that is easier to feel in terms of its effect on our emotions is stir-fried vegetables. The intense heat and quick movement adds energy to this dish. This becomes more intense if we add some grated ginger, garlic, and cilantro. When I eat this dish, I notice a warmth spread to my skin; at the same time, my emotions seem to come to the surface. I feel more expressive. I can make this sensation more apparent if I put some stronger spices into the dish.

What we are experiencing here is that certain ingredients, along with the way they're cooked, actually have a subtle influence on our emotions. It is not so strong that we cannot overcome the influence or that we lose self-control, but it is enough to make a difference when we need help to feel a certain way.

Comfort Foods

One way we use food emotionally is for comfort. We sometimes look to change an empty, hollow emotional feeling using food. Using food as a remedy in this way is a substitute for taking on the real challenge of working out why we have those feelings and exploring what kinds of transformation we would need to bring about to experience lasting changes. One of the problems with this is that we can get into a cycle where we use food to fill an emotional gap, but the food we're using is actually contributing to the problem because it is high in added sugar and upsets our blood sugar, precipitating further emotional highs and lows.

Comfort foods are usually sweet, creamy, and filling. For me, the ultimate comfort food is tiramisu, which has all these qualities. However, I can use this experience to explore other foods that might serve the same purpose. I find that stewed fruit has similar qualities in that it is sweet, has a creamy texture, and is filling. If I wanted to make it richer, I could add some natural yogurt or fresh organic cream.

For some people, a puréed pumpkin or root vegetable soup will be sweet and creamy enough. Here, you could add some olive oil to make it richer. If you need something even richer, you could try deep-fried vegetables or sauces made from tahini or nut butters.

By including a variety of these foods in your diet, you can reduce your desire for sugary foods while you engage in your own journey of change using the processes of awareness you have learned in this book.

Calming Foods

There may be times when we want to feel calmer and perhaps find it easier to meditate on our breathing and access our deeper feelings. During these times it's especially important not to consume any strong stimulants. In addition, I would suggest that a diet that includes more vegetables than any other type of food will help. Vegetables have a light, fresh, watery quality that can help our own energies move freely, with the result that we feel more peaceful. This is especially true when the vegetables are raw, steamed, boiled, stewed, pressed, pickled, or in a soup rather than fried, grilled, roasted, or baked.

You might also find that eating more fruit helps you feel calmer. Again, raw, steamed, or stewed would be better. Various herb teas can have a calming quality, especially when used to replace coffee or a caffeine-rich tea like English Breakfast tea. In macrobiotic thinking, there are some special items that are considered to be calming and were originally used by Zen monks. These are grated daikon (also known as mooli), kudzu, tofu, green tea, and shiitake mushrooms.

Daikon is a long, white radish. You can use other types of radishes as an alternative. Traditionally, daikon was grated and mixed with a few drop of shoyu (soy sauce), or grated and added to green tea or kukicha (Japanese twig tea).

This acts as a blood thinner and is considered to dissolve fats in the body. In terms of emotions, in my experience it helps me feel as though my emotions are slightly more dispersed.

Kudzu is made from a strong root vegetable that grows deep into the ground. Kudzu (also spelled kuzu) is sold in packets in the form of a chalky white powder. It is heated up in liquids to make them thicker. When combined with hot apple juice, it makes a relaxing drink that I have found can help calm my mind.

In Chinese medicine, tofu is considered a cooling food; I find it helps me feel lighter compared to comparable foods like cheese, fish, or meat. Tofu is best steamed, boiled, or used in soup to enhance its calming quality. In my experience, fried tofu has the opposite effect and is stimulating.

Green tea is interesting, as it is high in caffeine but also contains a nutrient that inhibits the body's absorption of caffeine. In the East, it has the reputation of being calming. Personally, I do find it helps clear my head, but perhaps no more than chamomile, fresh mint, or sage tea.

Shiitake mushrooms have been shown to reduce cholesterol in the blood and, in macrobiotic thinking, also reduce other fats in the blood. These mushrooms can help me feel more tranquil. They are most commonly used in miso soups, where they can be combined with small cubes of tofu.

In my experience, these foods can help me feel slightly calmer and can alter my emotions; however, eating too much of them or having them too often can be weakening.

PRACTICAL EXERCISES

1. Try avoiding all alcohol, coffee, sugar, chocolate, and strong spices for a few days and note how you feel. Be aware of your emotions.
2. If you tend to reach out for comfort foods high in added sugar, try stewed fruit, pumpkin or root vegetable soups, deep-fried vegetables, and sauces made from tahini or but butters instead.
3. Experiment by eating various dishes and being aware of how you feel. See if certain dishes consistently help you feel a certain way. Try com-

paring salads and fresh fruit with soups, stews, and porridge. Make a spicy stir-fry and be aware of your feelings.

4. Experiment by eating a diet high in vegetables for a week. Include some daikon, kudzu and apple juice, green tea or other herb tea, and miso soup with tofu and shiitake mushrooms. Try your gentle breathing meditation and see if you find it easier to connect with your deeper self.

SUMMARY

1. Foods have their own energies, and when we eat a certain food, its energy has a subtle influence on ours. The result is that we might find it easier to experience certain emotions.

2. Strong stimulants such as alcohol, caffeine, and sugar can open our heart centers chaotically.

3. Alcohol has the effect of taking us out of our centers and, in effect, out of our bodies, minds, and hearts. This can be disruptive to our emotions.

4. Coffee can raise our adrenaline levels and put us in a state of fight or flight, where we feel stressed and irritable.

5. Coffee can overstimulate our minds, taking us away from feeling our heart centers and being intuitive.

6. Sugar and foods high on the glycemic index or load raise our blood sugar quickly, leading more intense emotions. The sugar high is often followed by a blood sugar low, when it can be easier to feel flat. At the same time, it's likely that we will experience cravings for sweets. All this distracts us from being in our centers and feeling our hearts.

7. All foods may have a subtle influence on our emotions. More obvious examples are salads and fruit compared with soups and stews or a spicy stir-fry.

8. When we eat whole living foods, we consume some of the living energy and this has an influence on our emotions.

9. Ingredients and cooking style combine to create the energy of a dish.

10. We sometimes use foods to fill an emotional void. These are known as comfort foods. If our comfort foods upset our blood sugar levels, then they could make the situation worse.

11. Try substituting existing comfort foods with stewed fruit, thick pumpkin or root vegetable soups, deep-fried vegetables, and sauces made from tahini or nut butters.

12. Certain diets can be calming to our emotions and help us connect to our hearts and souls. Such diets could include plenty of vegetables—including salads and blanched, steamed, pickled and raw vegetables—along with some fruits and herb teas.

13. In Japan, a long white radish called daikon, a white chalky powder called kudzu, tofu, green tea, and shiitake mushrooms are all considered to help calm our emotions.

PART FOUR
HEALING THE BODY

In this section, we'll explore ways to heal our bodies. We'll start by learning how to test our bodies. How well do you know what's going on inside you? From there, we can try out different foods, exercises, stretches, chants, ways to care for our skin, and ways to sleep well. We'll explore the biology of our bodies and look at how to keep our physical beings in good shape. There is much here to use for the prevention of ill health and to help us live long lives.

CHAPTER TWENTY-ONE
Testing Our Bodies

Macrobiotic philosophy and lifestyle offers a unique approach to self-transformation. Macrobiotic practice may improve our energy, stamina, and flexibility, as well as our mental well-being and creativity. It also enhances intuitive, instinctual, and intellectual abilities and opens us up to greater levels of spiritual growth.

—MEMBERS OF THE INTERNATIONAL MACROBIOTIC ASSEMBLY

As I mentioned earlier, it's essential to have a feedback system to know where we are and whether we need to make adjustments. To have our own feedback system, it's helpful to use a range of indicators. Those I use on a regular basis are how well I can exercise, my pulse, how easily I can get to sleep, whether I can sleep well, my dreams, how easily I can meditate, my weight, my appetite, any food cravings, my bowel movements, the color of my urine, the condition of my skin, how often I suffer from minor illnesses, and my emotional state. The more familiar I am with my body and the better I know myself, the more aware I am at an early stage when I need to make adjustments to my diet and lifestyle. In theory, this helps me remain closer to my ideal state, without making large detours into feeling unhealthy before starting to make adjustments.

In this chapter, I've described a step-by-step approach to gaining greater awareness of ourselves so that we can more accurately sense how we are. The main aim of this chapter is to help you gain a greater awareness of yourself.

When learning to listen to your body, I suggest you just do that. Try not to give anything you feel a meaning or use it work out whether you're healthy or not. If you do this, you risk clouding and prejudicing your observations. Not only that, but once you start analyzing yourself, you move from your heart to your mind and reduce your ability to really feel.

I would also suggest that it's not healthy to use any of this information to compare yourself with other people. The sole use of becoming more aware is to help you feel your body—and not to use the awareness to boost your ego or become a hypochondriac.

LISTENING TO OUR BODIES

To listen to your body, I suggest you try this meditation: Lie down and make sure you're comfortable. Find that relaxing posture; put a cushion under your head or neck and, if it helps, under your knees. Start with the breathing meditation. Initiate every in and out breath while focusing your mind solely on your breathing. Once you feel centered and relaxed, focus on each part of your body. You can move a pair of imaginary hands around your body if it helps.

I suggest you visit each part of your body and ask questions, such as: Does this part of my body feel hot or cold? Light or heavy? Tired or energetic? Stiff or relaxed? Comfortable or painful? Take a journey from your toes to your head. Visit your feet, ankles, calves, knees, thighs, hips, abdomen, lower back, solar plexus, chest, upper back, shoulders, fingers, wrists, forearms, elbows, biceps, neck, jaw, teeth, nose, sinuses, eyes, ears, back of head, forehead, and crown. Spend a little time connecting with each place before moving on.

Each time you do this, you'll get to know yourself better; even the act of listening to each part of your body is healing in itself. This can then become your baseline for how you feel. Once you've established this as a reference, you can use it to measure how you feel after eating different foods or exposing yourself to various experiences and influences.

Another way to listen to your body is to do the gentle breathing meditation and be open to messages from your body. You can even use your ability to focus only on your breathing as a test of your current state. The more quickly you can get into a centered state and feel your own love, and the easier it is to maintain that state the more centered and calm your energetic body is.

Energy

Human energy is the result of mixing our food with oxygen. The energy we have is a reflection of our breathing, our diets, our metabolisms, and how we process energy. It helps to be aware of our energy levels so that we can reflect on these functions.

The easiest way to measure energy is to exercise regularly, and see how easy it is to complete a task or how long you can exercise for. I do forty minutes on a cross trainer, go swimming, and take long walks to exercise; doing each of these tells me more about my condition that day.

Make a note of how consistent your energy is in a typical day. When do you feel tired? Is there a repeating pattern?

Pulse

Your pulse provides useful feedback on the state of your heart and circulatory system. Take your resting pulse a few times in a typical day and see how it changes depending on your emotional state. You could also take your pulse before eating and half an hour afterwards to see how different meals affect your pulse. Take your pulse while exercising to find out its peak, fastest rate. When you finish exercising, time how long it takes for your pulse to return to its normal resting rate.

The easiest way to take your own pulse is to place the back of one wrist in the palm of your other hand. Let the fingers of the other hand bend around the wrist of the first hand so they reach over a small bone in the wrist below the thumb joint. Now you can move the tips of your fingers around until you feel your pulse.

You may notice that your pulse feels different at different times. Sometimes it may be soft, other times it might feel smooth, and another time hard and almost hammering. Sometimes you will feel your pulse on the surface and at other times you may need to press down a little to find it.

Sleep

Deep sleep is essential for good health, as it's during sleep that we repair our cells, DNA and energetic bodies. During our deep sleep our pineal glands secrete melatonin, which is a powerful antioxidant used to repair the body. This is effective only when we're in a state of complete rest.

Make a note of when you go to sleep and how easy it is to fall asleep. Be aware of how well you sleep. Do you have to get up during the night to urinate? If so, is this affected by how much you drink, whether you drink late in the evening, or by consuming coffee? Can you wake easily, and how do you feel in the morning? Do you have a sleep routine where you fall asleep and wake up more or less at the same time every day?

It's also interesting to be aware of your dreams. Do you have disturbing dreams and, if so, do they share a theme? Do your dreams wake you up? Can you remember them? Be aware of any correlation there may be between your dreams and your diet, emotions, and events in your life. I've noticed that after eating fish I sometimes have dreams of a more violent nature.

Appetite

Our appetites can tell us a lot about our diets, the state of our digestive systems, and emotional associations with food. We may experience a huge appetite and desire to feel full to compensate for certain emotions that we don't enjoy. At times of poor health, our bodies may naturally reduce our appetites to allow us to focus our resources on healing. It's common to use food to help trigger emotions. That midmorning coffee and cookie, afternoon piece of cake, or evening chocolate can all provide clues to how we might want to explore emotional issues or find better ways to maintain more consistent blood sugar levels.

In addition, strong cravings for food might occur when we are nutritionally deficient, as our body tries to get us to fill nutritional gaps. Temporary cravings can therefore be a sign that we need more of a certain type of food. This is most common when seasons change and our bodies want us to change our diets.

For now, the task is to be aware of your appetite. You might find it helpful to note in your diary when you crave certain foods. Be aware if your appetite increases at certain times of the day, and when you have cravings for certain foods. Do you feel satisfied after a meal? Do you eat certain foods when feeling stressed? Do you have temporary cravings that could reflect a nutritional deficiency? Do you feel a need to change your diet as the seasons change?

Another aspect of appetite is our sexual appetite. You could make a note of your sexual vitality and see how this is influenced by your emotions. How is your sexual appetite affected by stress? Do certain foods act as aphrodisiacs?

You could also consider your appetite for life. How strong is your desire to make the most of the rest of your life? Are you happy to drift along and just do what's necessary? Is this fairly consistent, or do you have days when you feel like you want to do the most you can with your life and others when you can't be bothered?

Weight

We live in an age when body fat has become a big issue, and the reason many people become interested in macrobiotics initially is to lose weight. I would not recommend becoming obsessive about your weight, and if you have this tendency I recommend that you ignore this section.

I find it helpful to weigh myself and be aware of how my clothes fit me. It's interesting to me how certain foods put more weight and body fat on my body. I also like to see how different exercise regimes influence my weight. Essentially, our weight and size is a reflection of whether we use up the energy in our food through our normal activities.

To be aware of your weight, simply find a consistent time to weigh yourself. Your weight will fluctuate throughout the day. In theory, you should be most stable in terms of weight when you first wake up. I must stress that weighing yourself is just one piece of feedback, and if you have a goal to reach a certain weight you may create internal conflicts that make it harder to feel healthy.

It's currently popular to think of weight in terms of body mass index (BMI), which is used to gauge when someone is overweight or obese. To calculate your BMI, you divide your weight by your height multiplied by itself. In metric units, this would be your weight in kilograms divided by your height in meters squared. For example, I am 1.83 meters tall and my current weight is eighty kilograms. To find my BMI, I would divide eighty by 1.83 multiplied by 1.83. My BMI comes out to 23.9.

In U.S. units, BMI is calculated by multiplying your weight in pounds by 703 and then dividing by your height in inches squared. Measured this way, my BMI would be 176 pounds multiplied by 703 and then divided by seventy-two inches multiplied by seventy-two inches. This also comes out to 23.9. This is a very broad and crude measure, as it doesn't take into account differences in bone, muscle, or organ mass.

An alternative to weight or BMI is to use your clothing to get a general indication of whether you're creating more fat or using up some of your fat reserves.

Be aware of what weight or size feels comfortable to you. If you're engaging in a lot of strenuous physical exercise, your weight can actually increase while your size reduces, because the same volume of muscle weighs more than fat. So if you increase your overall muscle mass but burn off lots of fat, your relationship between your weight and size will change.

Bowel Movements

How regular are your bowel movements? Be aware of when and how often you have a bowel movement in a typical week or day. When you have bowel movement, be aware of whether your stools feel hard, soft, or loose. Make a mental note of their color and size.

To find out how long it takes food to move through your digestive system, eat some corn on the cob, making a point of swallowing the kernels whole. Note when you eat them. Keep checking your stools until you see that the corn kernels have passed through your digestive system. Note the time and calculate how long it has taken for the food to pass through your system.

Urination

There's a lot of controversy over how much water to drink in a typical day, with many people claiming we should drink two or even up to five pints (one to two and a half liters) each day. This is often based on research showing that typically a person loses about five pints per day. However, in working out how much water we need to drink, we would also need to know how much water we consume in our diet as well as how much fluid we take in from the air.

Typically, someone eating a diet that includes fruits and vegetables will consume five pints of water per day. Certainly anyone eating a diet with plenty of whole, natural foods along with some herbal tea will take in sufficient liquid. This is not to say that drinking a glass or two of water a day is not beneficial; however, forcing ourselves to drink excess water can also create challenges in terms of blood pressure as well as the load on our hearts and kidneys. Our fluid requirements also depend on the weather and how much we sweat during exercise.

The easiest way to tell whether you're drinking enough water is to be aware of how often you urinate and the color of your urine. If you urinate frequently and your urine has a clear appearance, you may be consuming too many liquids. If you urinate infrequently and your urine has a strong color and/or smell, you may not be drinking enough.

Make a note of when you urinate throughout the day and note your urine's color. You could use terms like clear, pale, or dark. Review this after a few days to see if there's anything you can learn in terms of how much liquid you could drink. Experiment with drinking more or less liquid and note the effect on your urine.

Bloating and Wind

Another way to assess the condition of your digestive system is to note whether you experience abdominal bloating, excessive wind, or discomfort. Sometimes we just put up with these ailments and persevere with the same old diet. I would recommend using these conditions as useful feedback to improve your diet.

The first step is to become aware of which foods cause the bloating, discomfort, or wind. To assess this, you could keep a food diary and note everything you eat and how you feel afterwards.

You could experiment with trying different dishes from what you normally eat to see if you can find foods that are easier to digest. You could try taking out certain foods to see how you feel. Foods that commonly aggravate these digestive conditions are yeasted breads, white pasta, carbonated drinks, whole grains, beans, dairy foods, meat, onions, cauliflower, cabbage, and broccoli.

Another area of research would be the difference between eating cooked foods and raw foods. If you feel better when your food is cooked, you could explore if it makes a difference to cook something a little longer.

Your own eating habits might make a big difference. Try eating after you've been seated and relaxed for a while. You could combine this with chewing each mouthful until your food is liquid. Keep taking note of how you feel.

Eating some fermented foods, such as pickles, with each meal can introduce the kinds of healthy bacteria that make digestion easier.

Once you get to the point where your digestion feels comfortable, try bringing back foods that used to cause a problem. Do this one at a time and once in a while, to see if you have now created the internal environment in your digestive system to digest them properly. This will tell you more about the current state of your intestines.

Acid and Alkaline Balance

Our body fluids can change in terms of whether they are acidic or alkaline. This is known as our pH balance. Our pH balance can change according to the foods we eat and our emotions. We look into this fully in Part Five.

We can find out what our pH balance generally is by using our saliva and urine as a guide. You can measure your saliva and urine by using pH sticks or strips. You can purchase these specifically for measuring saliva and urine. Ideally, the strips or sticks would have a range that includes readings between 5.5 and 8.0.

In the pH scale, 7 is neutral. Values above 7 are alkaline, and below, acidic. Ideally, you would have a general pH reading between 7.0 and 7.5. Many people I test are below 7.0, which would suggest an acidic condition. Our pH changes throughout the day; it's typical to get a more acidic reading at 2 a.m. and a more alkaline reading at 2 p.m.

To test your saliva, you need to find a time when you haven't consumed anything but water during the previous two hours. In the morning, before you brush your teeth, is ideal. For testing your urine, I would suggest you test the first time you urinate on a given day, as the following urine tends to be a reflection of what you previously ate or drank along with whether you've been feeling stressed.

To get a reasonably accurate reading, I would suggest you test your saliva and urine for two or three days. Alternatively, if you want a better indication of how your eating and emotions are influencing your pH levels, test yourself every morning and use this as an indication of whether your previous day's eating was acid- or alkaline-forming and whether you were feeling stressed.

Skin

Our skin breathes, and thus is one of our main organs for excreting waste. Various forms of waste drift out to and through our skin. Sometimes this upsets our skin, causing rashes, spots, or red patches. Another possibility is that our natural oils do not flow to our skin, leaving dry patches. Our skin will also be affected by poor circulation. In addition, our emotional energies filter out through our skin and so, in theory, our skin will reflect their condition. Strong emotions can be reflected in our skin, and consistent long-term emotions like stress can risk the health of our skin.

Try testing your skin for elasticity. Take a pinch of skin from your forearm or the top of your hand. Pull it and let go. Watch to see how quickly your skin returns to its normal state. Check your skin regularly and note any spots, dry patches, pimples, redness, or oily areas. Think about whether this corresponds with a period of stress or changes to your diet.

If you rub your body with a hot, damp cotton cloth, you may notice that some areas do not turn red. This is most likely to occur on your legs; it indicates areas where the blood circulation is not as good as in the areas that change color quickly.

Be aware of any tendency for your hands to feel clammy, or of any increased sweating. You can get further feedback by being aware of your body odors. I find that drinking coffee leads to sweating more easily, and that after coffee my sweat has a distinctive smell. I have also noticed that my skin sometimes takes on the smell of cheese if I eat too much of it.

Fingernails

Until recently, looking at the fingernails was considered a valid method of medical diagnosis. Even now, an older doctor might take the condition of your fingernails into account. The most common test is to press the nail of your index finger down firmly with the thumb of your other hand and then remove your thumb. The flesh under the nail will turn pale and then return to its normal color. The theory is that if it bounces back to its normal color quickly, your blood is in a healthy state. If it takes a longer time, you might be deficient in iron or other minerals.

Try this test from time to time so you get an idea of how quickly your flesh usually returns to its normal color; if you're feeling unusually tired, you can try the test again and see if it takes longer than normal to regain your natural color.

Elasticity

One measure of health is how elastic we are. We could apply this measure to our physical or mental health. As we age, there is a tendency for our bodies to lose flexibility. Bones can become brittle, muscles get stiffer, ligaments and tendons tighten, skin loosens, bloods vessels harden, and our thinking can become rigid.

It can therefore be helpful to be aware of how elastic we are and use this as an indication of our current state. If we stretch regularly, we will be aware when certain stretches feel difficult or when we cannot reach a certain position. We can use this to reflect on whether aspects of our diets and lifestyles are working against us. Do more saturated fats and excess salt lead to feeling stiffer? Does a period of stress cause our muscles to tighten? Are our working conditions leading to bad posture and stiffness? In our experience, is there any relationship between feeling physically stiff and being mentally rigid?

Emotions

Our general emotional states will further help us feel our current states. I would recommend being aware of our emotions to the extent that we know when we are in a period where our emotions have changed. It would also be interesting to explore whether any emotional change can be associated with a change in diet, lifestyle, or usual practices. We could then be aware of the extent to which meditation, exercise, and food—among other possible forces—influence our emotions.

Immune System

Another way we can assess our general health is through the effectiveness of our immune systems. If we suffer from minor illnesses regularly, we might conclude that our diets, lifestyles, or outlooks are not working for us as well as they could be. George Ohsawa allegedly purposefully exposed himself to various illnesses to demonstrate his ability to recover.

For some time, I used to suffer from three or four colds a year. It was only when I made a conscious effort to maintain a more alkaline condition that this dropped to only one or two cold a year, including one year without a single cold. The colds were a useful indication for me that there was room to improve my health, and eventually I found the adjustment I needed to bring this about.

To gauge the effectiveness of your immune system, be aware of how often you suffer from a sore throat, a cold, the flu, a stomach upset, ulcers, warts, and similar immune-related illnesses. In addition, be aware of how long it takes you to recover. Similarly, you could note how long it takes to heal a cut. We'll explore ways to work with our immune systems in Chapter Thirty.

PRACTICAL EXERCISES

1. Lie down and go into your breathing meditation. Once relaxed, start to explore every part of your body, being attentive to your feelings. Try this daily so that you become aware of how your body changes from one day to the next.
2. Exercise regularly, and use it to create an awareness of your current condition.
3. Get to know your pulse rate, and try taking your pulse before, during, and after exercise. See how long it takes your pulse to return to its resting rate after exercise. Try taking your pulse before and a little while after eating.
4. Use your sleeping patterns to get useful feedback on your current state. Be aware of whether you get a full night's sleep without interruptions. Note any dreams, and see if they reflect your current emotional state.
5. Be aware of any strong cravings for food. Try to feel where the craving is coming from and how you could best address it.
6. Be aware of your sexual appetite and of any nutritional, emotional, or other factors that play a part in your sexual vitality.
7. Be aware of how your general appetite for life changes through different periods.
8. If appropriate, be aware of your weight or size, and use it to gauge whether your diet is in some kind of balance with your lifestyle, exercise, and other activities.

9. Be aware of your digestion and how your body feels after eating; and use your awareness to how different meals and your eating habits affect your digestion.

10. Use your bowel movements to gain further feedback on your food. Find out how long it takes food to pass through your digestive system by swallowing whole corn kernels whole and observing how long it takes them to appear in your stools.

11. Observe the frequency of urination and the color of your urine to get feedback on whether you're drinking the amount of fluids that's right for you.

12. Be aware of any bloating or wind, and use this to reflect on your food, cooking, and chewing.

13. Use pH strips or sticks to measure the alkalinity/acidity of your saliva and urine. Keep a record and be aware of what kind of foods and emotions affect your pH balance.

14. Be aware of the condition of your skin; try testing it for elasticity by pulling and releasing the skin on the top of your hands.

15. Be aware of any increase in sweating and whether the smells of your body change after eating certain foods. Make a note of any tendency for your palms to become clammy.

16. Try pressing on your fingernails and observe how quickly the flesh underneath returns to its normal color. Try this test if you feel weak or tired, and see if it takes longer for the flesh under your fingernails to return to its normal color.

17. Develop a stretching routine to help you be aware of how elastic you are. Be aware of any changes in stiffness, and see if you can relate this to changes in diet, emotions, or lifestyle.

18. Be aware of your emotional state and explore why you might take on certain moods.

19. Keep track of how often you become ill and use this as a measure of how strong your immune system is.

SUMMARY

1. It's essential to have a feedback system to know where we are in terms of our health, so we can determine what adjustments we might need to make to our diets, lifestyles, and attitudes about life.

2. Being aware of our bodies and being able to listen to them provides the basis for a feedback system.

3. It's important to be aware without making comparisons to others or using our awareness to become obsessed with the state of our health.

4. One way to listen to our bodies is to lie down, relax, and feel each body part.

5. We can use exercise as a means to measure our energy levels.

6. Regularly taking our pulse will help us know our resting state. We can then use this as a reference for comparing our pulse during and after exercise, or after a meal.

7. Sleep is an essential part of healing and maintaining good health. We can use our sleep to be aware of our health. This would include the times we fall asleep and wake up, whether we have to get up during the night, and our dreams.

8. Our appetites can tell us a lot about our emotional associations with food, whether we use food to suppress emotions, and whether we're going through a period nutritional deficiency.

9. Our sexual vitality could provide more clues to the current state of our health.

10. Similarly, our appetites for life might reflect our current condition.

11. Our weights and sizes reflect whether there's a balance between the energy we take in through food and the energy we use during the day.

12. Currently, it's popular to calculate body mass index, but it would be simpler to be aware of how your clothes fit from one day to the next.

13. Muscle weighs more than the same volume of fat.

14. We can learn more about our diets through how they affect our digestion and, in particular, whether certain foods precipitate bloating, wind, or indigestion.

15. Our bowel movements and stools can provide useful feedback on the effects of our diets.

16. We can time how long food takes to travel through our digestive systems by swallowing whole kernels of corn.

17. The color of our urine and frequency of urination are a useful guide as to whether we're drinking too much or too little water.

18. We can measure the pH balance of our saliva and urine to get a general indication of whether our bodies are in an acidic or alkaline state.

19. Our skins are excretory organs that can provide feedback on our overall conditions. Dry or oily skin, along with pimples, spots, and rashes, can reflect our food and emotions. The elasticity of our skins provide further clues as to the state of our health.

20. Fingernails can be tested to assess whether our blood is low in minerals.

21. Stretching is a helpful way to measure our elasticity, which in itself is a useful guide as to whether our muscles are shortening and blood vessels hardening.

22. The number of colds, sore throats, and minor illnesses we get in a year provides helpful feedback on how effective our immune systems are.

CHAPTER TWENTY-TWO
Creating a Healthy Digestive System

I got acquainted with macrobiotics thirty-one years ago when I was seventeen, then a high school student, and it totally changed my life. The concepts of connectedness between all phenomena, the possibility of achieving absolute freedom and justice, as stated by George Ohsawa, were mind-blowing and made me see life in a totally different and exciting way.

I also loved the diet, which made me feel much more vital, rooted, and clear-minded. The changes I went through after starting to practice macrobiotics were so dramatic that I decided to move to Boston and study with Michio Kushi.

Together with Eugenia, my wife, I brought up four children this way, and I have taught macrobiotics to many people in many different places.

The world is very different now than it was in 1977, when I started, but I still feel that the underlying principles of the macrobiotic philosophy are as valid as they were then—probably more so, given the incredible and global challenges that we are facing on all levels of life.

—FRANCISCO (CHICO) VARATOJO, macrobiotic teacher, author, and consultant, and director of the Macrobiotic Institute of Portugal

Our digestive systems take in food, break it down, and turn it into a liquid from which we absorb nutrients. Nutrients are absorbed into our blood and processed in our livers. Water is then extracted from the waste, which is stored until we can eliminate it. This process was explained fully in Chapter Four.

We are blessed with amazing digestive systems that allow us to eat an extraordinary range of foods. Only rats come close. Like anything, our digestive systems do have their limits, and long-term abuse can compromise their health.

Ultimately, an inappropriate diet for our digestive systems can lead to bloating, wind, constipation, diarrhea, pains, ulcers, and, eventually, more serious complaints such as diverticulitis, irritable bowel syndrome, stomach cancer, and colon cancer. Generally, a diet that is high in fiber and contains helpful bacteria will encourage a healthy digestive system, whereas foods that are high in saturated fats and refined sugars, or foods that are highly acidic, can, if eaten in excess, damage our digestive systems.

Our digestive systems rely on a delicate balance of acids, alkaline juices, enzymes, bile, and bacteria to work efficiently. Some foods move through our digestive systems slowly, while others pass through quickly. Slow-moving foods such as meat can putrefy and coat the intestinal lining with fat, encouraging toxins to build up.

Through your own awareness of our digestive systems and by listening to our bodies as we explore different foods and ways of eating, we can start to be aware of which of the following thoughts apply to us.

FIBER

There are two broad types of fiber: soluble and insoluble. Soluble fiber helps lower blood cholesterol and helps control blood sugar. This type of fiber is found inside plant cells. Insoluble fiber helps move food through the digestive system, reduces the risk of constipation, and cleanses the intestines. This type of fiber is concentrated in plants' cell walls.

In addition, it is thought that high-fiber foods help with weight loss, due to their greater bulk and ability to help us feel satisfied for longer. Edible fiber is also thought to clean our intestines, as the roughage has a slightly abrasive effect, helping to prevent any buildup of fats on our intestinal walls.

Insoluble fiber in our diets bulks up our stools, helping to prevent constipation and leading to more healthy bowel movements. It is not what we absorb but what we eat and do not absorb that determines the colon's internal condition.

Vegetables, fruits, whole grains, beans, nuts, seeds, and sea vegetables tend to be our best sources of dietary fiber. It helps to eat the edible skins of fruit and vegetables. Fish, meat, and dairy foods are low in fiber. Meat, eggs, and dairy foods are high in saturated fats.

FERMENTED FOODS

At the beginning of the 1900s, Nobel Prize–winning Russian bacteriologist Elie Metchnikoff explored the possible benefits eating fermented foods. He noticed that Bulgarians had an average lifespan of eighty-seven years and, later, that the Hunzas of Kashmir and the Georgians enjoyed an amazing history of longevity. He noted these cultures regularly consumed sour milks fermented using active lactobacilli bacteria.

In 1935, certain strains of *Lactobacillus acidophilus* were found to be very active when living in the human digestive tract. Further research has found that there are great health benefits to establishing a balance of good bacteria in the gastrointestinal tract through consuming friendly bacteria. Potential improvements include good digestion, a stronger immune system, and better detoxification.

Natural lacto-fermentation involves creating conditions in which naturally occurring organisms thrive and proliferate. By eating a variety of live, fermented foods, we encourage diversity among microbiological cultures in our bodies. This exposes us to a variety of potentially helpful microorganisms.

Foods that have these properties include miso, a fermented soybean paste; sauerkraut, pickled cabbage; pickles, vegetables that have been fermented in brine (salt water); gherkins, pickles made from a small variety of cucumber that often include some honey for flavoring; live yogurt, unpasteurized fermented milk; shoyu, a liquid made from fermented soybeans; natto, a fermented preparation of soft soybeans in a sticky paste; kimchi (sometimes spelled kimchee), spicy pickled Chinese cabbage; and tempeh, another version of fermented soybeans, prepared as a soft cake.

When buying any fermented food, make sure that you buy a version that is unpasteurized if you want to benefit from the action of fermentation and the living microorganisms. Also to get the benefit of these microorganisms, it's important to store the food in its ideal conditions before you eat it. The fermenting action and microorganisms are temperature-sensitive: too low a temperature and the activity ceases, and too high a temperature and the microorganisms die off.

The refrigerator is generally too cold for fermentation. If we eat fermented foods straight from the fridge, we are unlikely to experience any benefit. For example, yogurt would need to be at room temperature, actively fermenting, and tasting as though it might soon go bad in order to be effective at changing the environment in our digestive systems.

Foods that are pickled in brine or salt—such as miso, sauerkraut, pickles, gherkins, and shoyu—can be stored at room temperature as long as you eat them regularly. All that happens is that they continue fermenting. Eventually, after several months, they will taste excessively salty or too sour. In hot climates and in the summer you may want to find a cool place to store these foods, such as a dark cupboard.

Foods such as yogurt, natto, and tempeh can either be kept at room temperature and eaten within a few hours, or stored in the fridge and then left at room temperature for a few hours to encourage the fermentation to become active again before eating.

These foods can all be eaten warm, but if they exceed certain temperatures the microorganisms will not survive. Normally, sauerkraut, pickles, gherkins, yogurt, and natto are eaten at room temperature. However, it is common to cook miso, shoyu, and tempeh. I would suggest that, if you want to get the maximum benefit from any microorganisms, you add shoyu to a dish after it has been cooked and cooled down. Similarly, when you make a soup, portion it into bowls and then add the miso once the soup has cooled. Alternatively, you could use the miso to make sauces without cooking. Tempeh is more difficult to eat raw, as it tastes better fried or cooked into a stew; perhaps for this reason we could enjoy tempeh for its other qualities.

RAW FOODS

Raw foods are another source of healthy microorganisms. Research conducted on raw onions, scallions, leafy greens, artichokes, watercress, and leeks indicates that the microorganisms present on raw vegetables create far more healthy bacteria in the human digestive system than any probiotic nutritional supplement. This would suggest that regular consumption of raw vegetables will aid our digestive systems and help create a beneficial internal environment.

Raw foods could include salads or garnishes such as parsley or chopped scallions added to cooked dishes. It is common in southern European cultures to eat diced raw onion and slices of tomato with olive oil. This can be served as a side dish or put on top of grains or bean dishes. To expose my digestive system to the potential benefits of microorganisms, I try to eat some raw foods every day. It would help not to wash organic vegetables or, if you do rinse them, to leave them out for a while so that the microorganisms can become active.

SPEED OF DIGESTION

Different nutrients tend to pass through our digestive systems at different speeds. Generally, high-fiber foods tend to flow through more quickly, while foods high in saturated fats take longer.

According to this theory, fruits and vegetables would pass through our digestive systems more quickly than cheese or meat. Combining these foods can, in some people, lead to incomplete digestion, loose bowel movements, or bloating. For this reason you might find that your digestive system works better by, for example, eating fruits and meat at different times of day. Here you might have some fruit between meals rather than right after a meal.

Food Combining

Some people also find that they enjoy more comfortable digestion when they separate their consumption of grains from eggs, meat, cheese, or fish. This is known as food combining. Following this approach, lunch might consist of fish and vegetables and dinner of grains, beans, and vegetables. This way, the fish is not eaten with any grains.

Not everyone is affected by food combining; you can experiment by following the food combining pattern of eating for a few days to see if it makes any difference to how you feel after a meal.

Stomach Acidity

Some foods are acidic, and these can increase the acidity of our stomachs. However, these foods are not necessarily the same as acid-forming foods. We will explore this further in Chapter Thirty-five.

An overconsumption of acidic foods over a long period of time can, in some people, inflame the stomach lining, increase the risk of stomach ulcers, and lead to indigestion.

Examples of acidic foods are alcohol, coffee, citrus fruits, and foods high in sugar. In addition, it is thought that meat increases stomach acidity, as we produce more acids in order to digest it. The acidity created by these foods can be neutralized by consuming an alkaline food, such as vegetable juice, herb tea, or *umeboshi*, just before or after. For example drinking a glass of fresh vegetable juice before coffee would lessen the acidic effect of the coffee.

Through greater awareness of the feeling in your stomach after eating these foods, you can learn whether acidic foods adversely affect you.

Drinking

Drinking during or close to a meal can dilute our digestive juices, making it harder to digest our food properly. Again, this does not apply to everyone; you may need to experiment to find out to what extent you are influenced.

In addition, drinking a liquid that contains nutrients—such as the broth in a soup, juice, wine, or herb tea—may fill our stomachs for a longer time than liquids without nutrients, as we hold the liquid in our stomachs while we break down its nutrients. This can help us feel full, satisfied, and satiated for longer, as our expanded stomach presses on nerve endings that send messages to the brain that produce satiated feelings.

Breathing

We can breathe into our chests or into our abdomens, or both. If you place one hand over your chest and the other over your navel, you can feel whether your chest or abdomen moves most when you breathe.

If you can breathe into your abdomen, you'll massage the upper portion of your intestines with your diaphragm. To do this, make a conscious effort to pull your abdomen in as your breath goes out, and push it out as you breathe in. If you're not used to breathing into your abdomen, this can feel strange to begin with; you may need to practice several times a day until you feel you can naturally adopt this style of breathing. Massaging your abdomen through breathing can help you move food through your digestive system more easily and reduce the risk of food stagnating there.

Exercise

Walking and stretching can both aid digestion by physically helping to move food through our intestines. As we walk, we massage our ascending and descending colons with each step; this can have the beneficial effect of aiding the peristaltic action of moving food along.

Gentle abdominal stretches can also help. Standing up and stretching slowly to the left and right will move our ascending and descending colons. You can try this lying on your stomach or side to make it more relaxing. Slowly leaning backward and then forward will move our entire intestines.

After we eat, we send blood to our intestines to aid in the process of digestion and nutrient absorption. For this reason, you may find that strenuous exercise soon after a meal interferes with the digestive process, as exercise redirects some of your blood to your muscles.

Posture

Our digestive system is clearly arranged so that gravity helps in the process of moving food through it. Basically, we put food in near the top of our bodies and waste comes out near the bottom of our torsos. Many people through the ages have made the claim that sitting up straight during and after a meal aids our digestion and reduces the risk of ailments within the digestive system. I suggest you try sitting up straight during a meal and remain upright for some time after; see if you notice whether you're digesting more easily and comfortably.

Chewing

Chewing breaks down our food physically so that we can further break it down chemically in our stomachs. The more we chew, the more we expose the surfaces of the food to our digestive juices. If we swallow a lump of food, it will take longer for the liquids in our stomach to reach the center of that lump. In addition, our saliva chemically breaks down carbohydrates. This is why foods rich in carbohydrates, such as vegetables and grains, taste sweeter after they have been in our mouths for a while.

Try chewing your food until it feels like a liquid in your mouth. This might take thirty, forty, fifty chews—or more, depending on the food. When you do this, be aware of how much you need to eat to feel satisfied, and what effect it has on your digestion. Make a note as to whether chewing well has any influence on your desire for snacks between meals.

You may find that food tends to slip down your throat as you chew; you may have to make a conscious effort to keep your food toward the front of your mouth.

Eating Slowly

Eating slowly and drawing your meal out over a longer time can help the digestive process. It can be fun to make the meal a celebration or your evening's entertainment rather than rushing through your meal to go and do something else. When our lunch or dinner becomes our source of pleasure, we can take several hours gently eating while having fun with friends.

EMOTIONS

Our bodies are arranged so that in times of extreme fear or anxiety we eliminate all food from our digestive systems; this leaves us in the best physical shape to escape from danger and/or defend ourselves. This means that when we become stressed, anxious, or mildly fearful, our body is not ideally set up to receive food, or digest and absorb it. Some people will find their appetite reduces accordingly when they're under stress.

However, it's also possible that in an effort to get rid of the stressful feeling, we seek to replace it with feeling full and satisfied; thus some people overeat while feeling stressed. Although this is understandable from an emotional and energetic viewpoint, in the long term it may not be healthy, as we are working against our bodies' natural instincts and eating while we're not ideally prepared for digestion.

I would recommend trying to calm yourself before eating by using the breathing meditation, saying a prayer, or thinking of something that helps you relax. During a meal, watch a funny DVD, listen to music, laugh with friends, or read a romantic book to help remain calm and in a healthy state to accept your food.

One of the potential challenges with stress is that we tend to secrete more acid into our digestive systems and as a result risk becoming over-acidic. Over long periods of time, this can increase the risk of digestive disorders in some people.

A LITTLE DIRT CAN BE A GOOD THING

Small amounts of organic impurities might actually help make our digestive systems better able to resist ill health. The theory is that if our digestive systems are regularly challenged by small amounts of earth, then our immune systems become stronger and better able to deal with a major challenge such as food poisoning.

Whenever I'm cooking with organic root vegetables, I don't wash them unless there's obvious soil on their skins. Hopefully, small particles of earth will remain on the surface of the vegetables, mildly exercising my immune system. If your immune system is already weak or you're prone to upset stomachs, you'll need to approach this carefully, perhaps trying not washing the occasional vegetable, so that you don't overwhelm your immune system and instead slowly give it time to build up its strength.

PRACTICAL EXERCISES

1. Try eating only vegetables, grains, beans, fruits, nuts, and seeds for three days; note any change in your digestion and bowel movements.

2. Make a point of consuming some miso, sauerkraut, pickles, gherkins, live yogurt, kimchi, shoyu, or natto at every meal for a month, and see if you can feel any change in the state of your digestive system. Make sure you store and prepare these fermented foods so that the microorganisms are alive when you eat them.

3. Make a point of eating some raw vegetables with every meal for a week, and be aware of any changes to your digestive system.

4. Experiment with eating fruit only between meals for a month; be aware of whether this makes any difference to feelings of bloating, wind, or digestion problems.

5. For a week, try not eating grains at the same meal as fish, meat, or dairy foods; be aware of whether this has any effect on bloating, wind, or digestive discomforts.

6. Try a week without any alcohol, coffee, citrus fruits, meat, and foods high in sugar. Note the effects on your stomach, and then also note the feelings in your stomach when you bring them back.

7. For at least five minutes a day for a month, practice breathing so that you pull your abdomen in when breathing out and let your abdomen expand as you breathe in. See if this style of breathing can become your natural mode of breathing over time; be aware of any effect it has on your intestines.

8. Make a point of going for a walk or doing some light abdominal stretching about an hour after eating, and be aware of whether this helps your abdomen feel more comfortable.

9. Sit up straight at every meal for a week and be aware of any changes you feel.

10. During one meal, chew each mouthful of food at least thirty times, or until it feels like a liquid; be aware of how much you need to eat to feel satisfied.

11. Make a point of eating all your meals slowly for a week, and review how your digestive system feels.

12. Experiment with not washing organic vegetables for a month, so that you expose your digestive system to a little dirt.

SUMMARY

1. Our digestive systems break food down into liquids so we can absorb nutrients.

2. Although our digestive systems are incredibly versatile, we can eventually harm them through long-term abuse.

3. Through an awareness of our digestive systems, we can feel what foods and diets best suit us.

4. There are two types of fiber, soluble and insoluble. These can help with cholesterol levels, blood sugar levels, bowel movements, and cleaning our intestines.

5. Foods high in fiber are vegetables, fruits, whole grains, beans, nuts, seeds, and sea vegetables.

6. Fermented foods containing lactobacilli bacteria contain microorganisms that can help grow helpful bacteria in our intestines.

7. Fermented foods include unpasteurized miso, sauerkraut, pickles, gherkins, live yogurt, shoyu, natto, kimchi, and tempeh.

8. To benefit from the living microorganisms in fermented foods, they need to warm up to room temperature and stay there for some time before being eaten.

9. These microorganisms will be destroyed by heating and cooking.

10. Raw foods are an effective way of introducing more healthy microorganisms into our intestines.

11. Different foods pass through our digestive systems at different speeds; it is thought that eating foods that digest quickly, such as fruit, at different times of day from meat or cheese, which digest slowly, can help digestion in some people.

12. Food combining theories suggest that some people experience better digestion by separating grains from fish, meat, eggs, and dairy foods.

13. Foods that are acidic can increase the acidity of the fluids in our stomach. Meat may also raise acidity, as we produce more digestive acids to break it down.

14. Drinking during or close to a meal can dilute the digestive juices and impair digestion in some people.

15. Breathing deep into our abdomens massages our intestines.

16. Mild exercise after a meal moves our intestines, aiding digestion.

17. Gravity plays a part in digestion, and sitting up straight during and after a meal can improve digestion.

18. Chewing prepares our food for digestion physically and chemically.

19. Eating slowly gives our digestive systems more time to digest properly.

20. Stress, anger, fear, anxiety, and similar emotions can create a state in which we do not digest our food well.

21. Small amounts of organic dirt can improve our digestive systems and strengthen our immunities from more serious and potentially dangerous bacteria.

CHAPTER TWENTY-THREE
Foods for Physical Well-Being

"So who am I?" The question occurs in our thinking, and most of our thinking is continuous chatter, dialogues we have with ourselves through language and its accompanying images.

While language is used for communication, language's main function is to create our reality. Take the city of New York. Where does it exist? It is geographically located in the United States of America. Yet New York and United States are labels or nouns that exist not in nature but in language. When an eagle flies between the United States and Canada, it does not carry a passport. To the eagle, the distinction of the two countries does not exist. So the label "New York" exists only in language, and only for humans. No other species would mistake the United States for something real.

All words exist on the language map, and are not inherent to the natural world. The map is not the territory.

Yet, another important quality of language is that it has a life of its own. It exists independently of any one person and has existed for thousands of years. Just as I did not invent the label "United States" but inherited it at birth, so we are born into a preexisting language.

So language is a map, or a tool: a tool of distinction and description that has nothing to do with any one of us individually, that we're born into, that we use to navigate this world during our human existence.

Another quality of language is that it separates. This person, the separate self with which each of us identifies, is also just a linguistic distinction. What we think of as ourselves exist only in language, and as with all linguistic distinctions, is only a label. Take time to think about everything that you think you are, and you will see that all of it is described by language. Because we constantly talk to ourselves, our perception of ourselves appears to be material and real. What we fail to see is that these separate selves that we think we are do not exist in nature. Our "true natures" cannot be described by words, nor can they ever be thought.

In 2005, when driving my truck, I discovered how to stop the constant mental chatter that had accompanied my every waking moment. When one stops the chatter, everything that one identifies with as a "me" completely disappears. The separate self never existed.

—NORIO KUSHI, founder of demystifyingenlightenment.org

SHARING INSIGHTS INTO THE HUMAN CONDITION

In addition to digestion, the food we eat is influential on the basic biological and chemical functions of our bodies. This can ultimately affect every function of our bodies.

We inhabit amazing bodies that can function through incredible ranges of environments, including severe hardship and great deprivation. That humans can survive so long eating poor diets while regularly self-abusing with alcohol, drugs, and cigarettes just shows how resilient we can be. However, if we want to keep ourselves in optimum physical condition, we can use food to help ensure everything is working well. Once we accept that food is an important part of feeling well, the big question becomes: what is a healthy diet?

Unfortunately, there are so many diets, so much conflicting advice, and so much confusing research that what might have been a simple question has, for many, become a fear of not getting enough omega-3 fatty acids or of getting too many free radicals.

The macrobiotic approach has been to look at societies around the world that have enjoyed long periods of good health and longevity, and see what they have in common. We can also think about what we eat food for. Our food is essentially there to provide energy and nutrients that give us the ability to grow, repair our cells, and keep our internal environments functioning properly.

Healthy Societies

People from Okinawa, made up of the Japanese islands of Ryūkyū are thought to have the world's longest life expectancy. This has been attributed partly to the local diet. Compared to the mainland Japanese diet, the traditional diet of the islanders is twenty percent lower in calories and contains three times more green and yellow vegetables, particularly sweet potatoes. The traditional Okinawan diet is also low in fat and has only a quarter of the sugar and three quarters of the grains of the average Japanese diet, and it includes half a serving of fish a day and more fermented foods made from soy and other beans than the mainland's diet. Okinawans eat almost no meat, eggs, or dairy products. In theory, this would make theirs an alkaline-forming diet. Reportedly, the typical Okinawan reaching age 110 has had a BMI of 20.4 and a diet consistently averaging no more than one calorie per gram of food. Generally, foods range from 0.8 to 9.0 calories per gram—so this is very low.

The energy and endurance of the Hunzas living in the mountains of Pakistan could have as much to with what they don't eat as what they do. They consume about half the protein, one-third the fat, but about the same amount of carbohydrates as the average American. The carbohydrates that the people of Hunza eat are mostly unrefined, coming from vegetables, whole grains, and fruit instead of sugar and refined flour. The Hunzas eat little processed food, as most of their foods are fresh and in their original, unsalted state. Processing includes drying some fresh fruits in the sun and fermenting milk to make butter and cheese. The food is essentially organic.

Other areas of the world noted for longevity are parts of rural France and rural China, as well as those close to the Mediterranean Sea. Common dietary themes in all these societies are a high consumption of vegetables and fruits, and fewer processed grains. In the European regions, there is a high use of olive oil. Fish is a strong component of the Okinawan and Mediterranean diets. Fermented milk products feature in the Hunza and French cuisine.

Following this path, we could generalize that eating a diet high in vegetables, fruits, and beans, along with good-quality natural grains, fish, and olive oil, as well as some fermented foods, would form the basis of a healthy diet.

To gain another understanding of food, we can explore it from a modern nutritional perspective. This can be a useful complement to other ways we understand food, but in my opinion it is not a reliable basis for all of our food choices. I have included some of the commonly accepted and current ideas on nutrition here so we can explore another perspective.

ENERGY

One of the biggest roles of our food is to provide us with energy. The potential energy in food is measured in calories. Most of our calories are used to maintain the correct blood temperature so that various biological processes can take place. It's as though we burn the food with the oxygen we breathe in to create heat. In addition, we use calories to fuel our bodies for movement and function.

From a nutritional perspective, there is interest in how many of our calories come from food that also contains fat compared with how many come from food that contains fiber, minerals, and vitamins. If our energy mainly comes from dairy foods, for example, we may not be able to process the associated high levels of fat, leading to an unhealthy buildup of fat in the body.

We can also explore what we take in with our fuel. Refined sugar is pure calories and does not contain any other nutrients. The challenge is to get our energy from foods that also contain nutrients that are essential for good health. If we take in more energy than we need in a day, we simply put on fat—so, following this logic, if the food we get our energy from is devoid of useful nutrients, we either become deficient in certain nutrients or have to eat more and take in too much energy. You could think of in terms of how many healthy nutrients you absorb per calorie of energy.

In addition, it's interesting to explore how quickly certain foods raise our blood sugar. Foods that raise our blood sugar quickly can give us a rush of energy, but excess calories will often be stored in the muscles and then turned into fat. Slow-burning foods, which raise our blood sugar slowly, can lead to a sustained rise in energy levels and provide greater stamina and endurance.

Vegetables, whole grains, beans, and fruit provide energy that is reasonably slow-burning, comes from a source low in fats, and includes a wide range of other essential nutrients.

GROWTH

Protein is the nutrient that enables us to grow. Everything that grows needs protein and contains protein. All natural foods therefore contain protein, including all unprocessed forms of plant-based food. It would be practically impossible to eat a natural-foods diet without getting sufficient protein. The only way a diet can be deficient in protein is if it is high in added sugar, as sugar does not contain any proteins.

Amino acids are the building blocks of protein. The human body needs a group of essential amino acids to remain in good health. Essential amino acids are those we need to consume through our diet, as our bodies cannot make them. Meat, fish, eggs, and dairy foods each contain all the essential amino acids, whereas grains, beans, vegetables, fruits, seeds, and nuts do not individually contain all the essential amino acids—but when a variety of them are eaten over the course a typical day, they can easily satisfy most people's protein requirements.

When different plant foods are eaten in the same day—for example, grains and beans or grains and nuts—they combine to provide all the essential amino acids. In addition, having small amounts of fish, eggs, meat, and dairy foods on a regular basis will further ensure that we take in all the essential amino acids. It is most important that children and teenagers receive adequate protein while they are growing.

REPAIR AND PROTECTION

Many nutrients help us repair and protect our bodies. In this section we will briefly look at fats, minerals, vitamins, phytonutrients, and antioxidants. This information is based on an evolving science, and, while interesting and helpful in increasing our general knowledge and awareness of food, it is not helpful to create a diet based on current nutritional information, as this will take you away from your intuition, heart, and soul, and will ultimately keep you from using your common sense.

The essential fatty acids known as omega-3s and omega-6s are used by the body to help control inflammation and have been shown to have a beneficial influence on our hearts and immune systems. Good sources of essential fatty acids include seafood, soybeans and fermented soybean products, sunflower oil (preferable consumed raw), sunflower seeds, pumpkin seeds, hemp seeds, and walnuts.

Foods high in fat can help us build up fat around our organs; in moderation, this helps protect the organs. Some body fat also acts as insulation, helping our bodies maintain a consistent temperature with less effort and using less energy.

Antioxidants are a relatively recent discovery; they are thought to protect us from potentially harmful free radicals. Free radicals are atoms or molecules containing unpaired electrons; too many free radicals in the body may increase the risk of cancer. It is thought that a diet high in antioxidants can slow the aging process and lead to longevity. The role of antioxidants may become more important, as we appear to be increasingly exposed to sources of free radicals. Colorful vegetables and fruits are thought to be high in phytochemicals that that can act as antioxidants. In addition, green tea, red wine, and dark chocolate may contain antioxidants. Our bodies also make their own antioxidants while we sleep, in the form of melatonin. This powerful antioxidant appears to be easily taken up and used while we are in a state of rest.

It is currently thought that seventeen minerals, listed below, are required to support our biochemical processes and ensure the health and optimum function of our cells.

Calcium from beans, green vegetables, nuts, seeds, and dairy foods builds bones, neutralizes acidity, clears toxins, improves muscles, aids the digestive system, and helps the bloodstream.

Chloride is used to produce hydrochloric acid in the stomach, and for cellular health. Salt is a common source of chloride.

Cobalt is a component of vitamin B12. See below for more information on B12. Sources of cobalt include fish, nuts, green leafy vegetables, and grains.

Copper acts as a catalyst in the formation of hemoglobin, the part of our blood that carries oxygen. It is considered a powerful antioxidant, removing free radicals, and is considered by some people to alleviate arthritis. Sources of copper include whole grains, beans, shellfish, dark chocolate, fruits (especially cherries), leafy green vegetables, nuts, meat, and tofu.

Fluoride aids in the formation of tooth enamel. Food sources include fish and other seafood. Depending where you live, there may be fluoride in your drinking water, and it is often found in toothpaste.

Iodine is used by our bodies to synthesize thyroid hormone. Too much thyroid hormone can be as harmful as too little. Sources of iodine include fish and other seafood, sea salt, and sea vegetables. It may also be present in eggs and dairy foods, depending on the animal feed, and root vegetables, if the soil contains iodine and the vegetables are not over washed or peeled.

Iron is required for the function of many proteins and enzymes, including hemoglobin, making it an essential mineral for our blood quality. In addition, the spin of electrons in an iron atom is affected by the earth's magnetic field; this may influence our senses of direction and health in terms of our own electromagnetic fields. Good sources of iron are fish, meat, eggs, beans, whole grains, leafy green vegetables, and sea vegetables. Some people do not absorb iron from plant sources as well as from animal sources, and some people require good sources of vitamin C to absorb iron. Phytates in whole grains and beans that have not been soaked can reduce our absorption of iron and zinc.

Magnesium helps maintain the function of our muscle and nervous systems, keeps our heart rhythms steady, supports our immune systems, and keeps our bones strong. It also has a role in regulating our blood sugar and blood pressure levels. It helps increase alkalinity. Green vegetables, beans, whole unrefined grains, nuts, and seeds are good sources of magnesium. Even hard drinking water contains this mineral.

Manganese has an antioxidant function and plays a role in our metabolism of carbohydrates, amino acids, and cholesterol. It is also thought to play a role in bone development and wound healing. Sources include soaked beans and whole grains, nuts, leafy green vegetables, and teas.

Molybdenum is a trace mineral that is thought to be essential for enzymes involved in the chemical transformations in the carbon, nitrogen, and sulfur cycles. Rich sources include whole grains, nuts, and animal products. Vegetables can be a good source, but much depends on the quality of the soil in which they are grown.

Nickel influences the amount of iron our bodies absorb from the foods we eat. It may also help in the formation of red blood cells. Sources of nickel include beans, whole grains, and nuts. Vegetables can be a good source, depending on the quality of the soil in which they are grown.

Phosphorus helps build strong bones and teeth, and forms genetic material, cell membranes, and many enzymes. Phosphorus is found in many protein-rich foods such as fish, beans, nuts, eggs, meat, dairy products, whole grains, potatoes, dried fruit, and garlic.

Potassium helps the kidneys function and plays a key role in the health of our hearts. Being an electrolyte, potassium aids our hearts and minds in sending electrical impulses throughout our bodies. It smoothes muscle contraction and maintains good health in our bones. The balance of potassium in our bodies depends on how much sodium (salt) we consume. An overconsumption of salt can deplete our reserves of potassium. Alcohol and coffee are thought to increase the amount of potassium we excrete through urine. We can absorb adequate levels of potassium from vegetables, fruits, and beans. Fish, meat, and dairy foods also contain potassium. Tomatoes and bananas are often cited as common sources.

Selenium is a trace mineral incorporated into proteins; it is an important antioxidant, helping prevent cell damage from free radicals. This may help prevent degenerative diseases such as cancer and heart disease, as well as strengthen our immune systems. Plant foods are a good source of selenium, but much depends on the levels of selenium in the soil in which they are grown. Selenium is particularly abundant in Brazil nuts, and it can also be found in whole unprocessed grains, nuts, fish, meat, and eggs.

Sodium is another electrolyte, and also important for creating an environment where electrical signals can rush through our bodies. Interestingly, these electric impulses are much faster than the messages sent through our nervous systems; they may be part of what we think of as our energetic bodies. Sodium has an influence on how much fluid we retain and on our blood pressure. It plays a role in muscle contraction and keeps minerals such as calcium soluble in our blood. It's also thought to stimulate our adrenal glands. Most people allegedly consume too much salt, and in some of these people this results in high blood pressure. Salt is lost through sweating.

Sulfur is found in all body tissues; it's particularly associated with the health of the skin, nails, and hair. It's also thought to help cleanse our blood and protect us against the buildup of toxins. Sources of sulfur include beans, fish, meat, eggs, and dairy products.

Zinc supports the activity of about 100 enzymes, and helps maintain a healthy immune system. It helps heal wounds, is needed for DNA synthesis, and maintains our sense of taste and smell. Phytates in whole grains and beans that have not been soaked can reduce our absorption of zinc. Foods high in zinc include shellfish, meat, whole grains, nuts, and seeds, especially pumpkin seeds.

Vitamin A is important for the health of our eyes and skin; it also plays an essential role in cell division and growth. It's also thought to improve the effectiveness of our immune systems, be an antioxidant, and reduce the risk of heart disease and cancer. Foods high in vitamin A include carrots, broccoli leaves, sweet potatoes, kale, pumpkin, cantaloupe melon, apricots, papaya, mangos, broccoli, squash, liver, eggs, and butter.

Vitamin B1's main role is in helping metabolize carbohydrates, making it essential for good digestion. It's also involved in maintaining the health of our nervous systems. Good sources are yeast, whole grains, asparagus, kale, cauliflower, potatoes, oranges, kidney beans, pork, and eggs.

Vitamin B2 aids in metabolizing respiratory proteins, fats, and carbohydrates. It is helpful for maintaining the health of our skin, nails, eyes, mouths, lips, and tongues. Good sources include yeast, mushrooms, yogurt, soybeans and soy products, almonds, asparagus, eggs, greens, broccoli, lettuce, and meat.

Vitamin B3 helps with blood circulation and the function of the nervous system. It helps metabolize proteins and carbohydrates. It's involved in the maintenance of healthy skin as well as the synthesis of sex hormones. Foods high in vitamin B3 include fish, meat, whole grains, nuts, seeds, and green vegetables.

Vitamin B5 metabolizes carbohydrates, proteins, and fats into useable energy. It's thought to support the function of the adrenal glands, possibly helping us deal with stress. Foods that are high in this vitamin include mushrooms, sunflower seeds, peanuts, split peas, soybeans, yogurt, corn, broccoli, squash, cauliflower, eggs, and strawberries.

Vitamin B6 performs a variety of functions, including protein metabolism, red blood cell metabolism and the efficient function of our nervous and immune systems. Vitamin B6 also helps maintain our blood sugar levels. Sources include avocados, tuna, bananas, whole grains, sardines, mackerel, beef, poultry, cabbage, sunflower seeds, soybeans, walnuts, lentils, and eggs

Vitamin B7 is used for the metabolism of carbohydrates and fats as well as to support adrenal function. It helps maintain a healthy nervous system. This vitamin is involved in maintaining healthy skin, hair, and nails. Foods high in vitamin B7 include whole grains, corn, avocados, broccoli, cauliflower, beans, mushrooms, nuts, eggs, and meat.

Vitamin B9 is required for the production of red blood cells, and it also assists with cell function, tissue growth, and the synthesis of DNA. It also helps metabolize proteins. Sources high in this vitamin are whole grains, leafy greens, asparagus, beans, peas, strawberries and nuts.

Note that the B vitamins above are generally found in whole grains. It is important to eat the whole grain as the vitamins are mainly found in the outer layer. In addition over cooking can destroy some of the B vitamins.

Vitamin B12 helps with the formation of red blood cells and the maintenance of a healthy nervous system. It's necessary for the synthesis of DNA during cell division. Anyone practicing a vegan version of macrobiotic eating needs to be aware that vitamin B12 is not found in adequate quantities in any plant food; if you're vegan, I would suggest that you consider B12 supplements. Clams and other shellfish are high in B12. Fish, meats, and eggs are also good sources.

Vitamin C is important in forming collagen, a protein that gives structure to blood vessels, muscles, cartilage, and bones. It helps maintain capillaries, bones, and teeth, and is thought to play a major role in repairing the tissue in our hearts. Vitamin C is also considered to be a powerful antioxidant. Foods high in vitamin C include red peppers, oranges, broccoli, kohlrabi, strawberries, cantaloupe, tomatoes, mangos, tangerines, cabbage, sweet potatoes, and white potatoes. Generally, all fruits and vegetables contain vitamin C.

Vitamin D can be produced when our bare skin is exposed to sunlight; for many people, a dietary source is also required to avoid deficiencies in winter or when not out in the sun enough. Vitamin D promotes calcium absorption, helping maintain strong bones. It also helps our immune function and reduces inflammation. Fish is generally considered the best source of vitamin D. Much smaller quantities can be found in meat, cheese, and eggs.

Vitamin E is considered a powerful antioxidant, protecting cells from damage. It also plays a role in the function of our immune systems, repairing our DNA and helping various metabolic processes along. Vegetable oils, nuts, green leafy vegetables (especially spinach), broccoli, kiwis, seeds, and nuts (especially almonds).

Vitamin K is considered essential to the process of forming blood clots, which stops bleeding. It's also involved in bone mineralization, regulation of cell growth, and prevention of osteoporosis. Green leafy vegetables, olive oil, broccoli, and cabbage are considered helpful sources of vitamin K.

It's worth noting that many vitamins are sensitive to high temperatures; you may find that eating a variety of raw foods in your everyday diet helps ensure that you benefit from a complete range of vitamins.

New research is investigating the role of phytonutrients, also known as phytochemicals. These are found in fruits and vegetables, and they appear to have an important role in maintaining good long-term health. They may play a part in reducing the risk of cancer, have anti-inflammatory properties, and be powerful antioxidants. Some of the phytonutrients may be harmed by processing and cooking, again suggesting that regular consumption of raw fruits and vegetables helps us absorb these potentially health-giving nutrients.

Phytochemicals are found in a wide range of natural whole foods, including vegetables, fruits, beans, whole grains, nuts, and seeds. Eating a wide range of natural foods—rather than relying on whatever is currently being hyped by the media as the latest superfood—will ensure adequate consumption of nutrients.

BALANCE

There are many ways in which our bodies maintain their own balance. Two important aspects of balance, and ones that have played a part in macrobiotic dietary practice since the work of Sagen Ishizuka, are the balance of acidity and alkalinity and the balance of sodium and potassium. Our bodies will go to great lengths to maintain an ideal balance, but over time an excessively acid-forming or sodium-rich diet will challenge our resources and eventually lead to deficiencies, as our mineral and vitamin reserves are depleted in an effort to restore balance.

In theory and in my experience, in order to maintain a slightly alkaline condition, half of our daily food needs to be vegetables and fruits. With a few exceptions, most other foods, including grains, beans, fish, nuts, and seeds, are acid-forming.

There are many sources of sodium, and often we consume more than we realize, as sodium is commonly added to processed foods. As long as we consume plenty of vegetables, fruit, and beans, we will enjoy rich sources of potassium.

Acid and alkaline are explored in more detail in Part Five.

FOODS THAT HARM

An excess of any nutrient can be potentially harmful. Even a food like brown rice could harmful if over consumed, as it would take the place of other foods with other essential nutrients and lead us to be overly acidic. More obvious foods that can harm us if eaten in excess over long periods of time are refined sugar, salt, polyunsaturated fats used in cooking, trans fats, and saturated fats.

As refined sugar contains only calories, it provides energy without any other essential nutrients. If we consume refined sugar, we then need other foods to get all the other essential nutrients; these other foods also come with calories, making us overconsume in terms of energy, risking the creation of too much fat. It's also thought that eating refined sugar can, in some people, result in a loss of minerals from the teeth and bones.

Too much sodium can upset our balance of how much fluid we retain and lead to an imbalance of potassium, resulting in muscular problems. In the past, a typical macrobiotic style of eating could be high in sodium, as sea salt, miso, shoyu, *umeboshi* (pickled plums), *ume* vinegar, *tekka* (a condiment made from miso, sesame oil, burdock, lotus root, carrot, and ginger), *shiso* sprinkle (a condiment made with dried leaves of the herb *shiso*), *gomasio* (sesame salt), sauerkraut, and pickles are all high in sodium. I would suggest that it's helpful to also use other seasonings such as herbs, lemon juice, orange juice, other fruit juices, pepper, and oils.

Polyunsaturated oils are a group of vegetables oils that contain more than one double bond in the molecules of the fatty acid. This makes them chemically unstable and prone to break down when heated or exposed to sunlight. Eating them results in free radicals being introduced to our body, which can increase the risk of degenerative illnesses. Oils that are high in polyunsaturated fat include sunflower oil, corn oil, safflower oil, and most vegetable oil blends. Oils high in polyunsaturated fat would best be used raw on food instead of in cooking. Olive oil, which is high in monounsaturated oil, would be better for frying and using in soups and stews. Butter would be better for baking and frying than polyunsaturated vegetable oils.

Trans fats are industrially manufactured hydrogenated fats, created by adding hydrogen atoms to plant oils. This process creates an oil that is used for commercial baking and in the junk food industry. Overconsumption of these fats has been implicated in an increased risk of heart disease, Alzheimer's disease, cancer, diabetes, and obesity.

An overconsumption of saturated fats can increase the fat content of our blood for extended periods if we don't use the fat by, for example, working outside in cold weather. Eventually this can cause us to build up fat in our organs and on the inside of our arteries, leading to a risk of high blood pressure and heart disease. These fats have also been implicated in excess weight and increased risk of strokes. Foods high in saturated fats include meat, eggs, and dairy products.

More recently, attention has been brought to the role of free radicals and their influence on our health. In chemical terms, free radicals are atoms, molecules, or ions with unpaired electrons. These unpaired electrons can be highly reactive and are associated with increased aging and degenerative disease. A common source of free radicals is fried foods and foods that have been processed at high temperatures. This included many commercial baked foods that use vegetable oils. The oils in beans, grains, nuts, and seeds can also be adversely affected by processes that use high temperatures.

We can also become exposed to free radicals through eating foods that have oxidized. Foods in their whole, natural state are protected from the outside environment by their skins. Once we remove the skin, grind up the foods, or process them into a liquid, there is a risk that without proper storage they will oxidize; when we eat oxidized foods, we may be introducing unhealthy chemicals into our bodies. For this reason, it's safest to eat foods that have come straight from the land rather than out of a factory.

WHAT IS THE IDEAL DIET?

There's probably a lot of sense in the old instruction to eat a little of everything. Certainly it's helpful to eat a wide variety of ingredients and experience a big range of cooking styles to ensure that we receive all the nutrients necessary for life. I would add that it's important to eat foods in their natural states, as I feel our health is now being challenged by mass production and the wealth of new food processing techniques. So, to eat a little of everything natural would suit me. By "natural" I mean straight from the land, with only the natural processing of grains into bread and pasta, fermentation, and the cold pressing of oils.

Logically, we could say an ideal diet for human consumption is high in vegetables; includes some whole, unprocessed grains; contains some animal foods; has fermented foods; includes raw vegetables and fruits; and is primarily made up of fresh, whole, natural foods. I would also claim that if our primary diet is made up of foods such as vegetables, fruits, grains, beans, nuts, seeds, fish, and fermented foods, that it would also be appropriate to include a little of anything else from time to time according to our needs at that moment.

I think of all this information as a starting point and, if you like, an opportunity to manually take over what we eat for a while so that we can experience a different diet and use this experience to develop the resources to discover what works best for each of us. Ultimately, it is for each of us to listen to our bodies, be aware of the influence food has on us, and develop our intuition to find what particular diet best suits us at any time.

PRACTICAL EXERCISES

I suggest you start with those that represent the biggest dietary change for you.

1. Try eating a diet without any refined sugar or refined grains like white bread or white pasta for a week, so you can experience getting your energy from foods that are also high in useful nutrients.

2. If you have not eaten any fish, meat, eggs, or dairy food for a time, try eating a small amount each day for a week to discover whether you feel any different.

3. Include some raw vegetables and, if appropriate, raw fruit every day for a month and be aware of any difference you feel in your health.

4. Try making about half your daily food vegetables, and be aware of any difference you experience in your general health.

5. Be aware of how often you use sodium-rich foods for seasoning, and substitute these with herbs, oils, spices, and natural seasonings that are low in sodium.

6. Try frying in olive oil rather than polyunsaturated oils for a month. Use butter instead of vegetable oil for baking.

7. Experiment with avoiding any processed foods that include hydrogenated oils for a month.

8. Avoid all foods with saturated fat for a month, so you can experience how you feel with less fat in your blood. This would mean avoiding meat, dairy foods, and eggs.

9. Try eating only natural, unprocessed foods for a week and be aware of how you feel.

SUMMARY

1. We can look at diets of societies that live the longest to get clues on what diets might work best for us. Studies indicate a diet high in vegetables, fruit, fish, fermented foods, whole grains, and that also includes raw fruits and vegetables, would be ideal.

2. Refined sugar provides energy without any other nutrients. The more our energy comes from refined sugar, the greater the risk of nutritional deficiencies or accumulating fat.

3. Some forms of energy raise our blood sugar more quickly, encouraging us to convert sugar into fat.

4. Protein is required for growth. Amino acids are the building blocks for protein; meats, fish, eggs, and dairy foods contain all the essential amino acids. We can also consume all the essential amino acids when we eat a variety of plant-based foods such as beans and grains.

5. A diet that contains all the necessary minerals, vitamins, essential fatty acids, antioxidants, and phytonutrients will help us maintain good health.

6. A diet high in vegetables and fruit will generally be alkaline-forming.

7. Moderating the use of sodium-rich foods can improve our sodium and potassium balance.

8. An excess of any one food can be unhealthy and lead to nutritional deficiencies.

9. Foods that have the potential to harm us include sugar, salt, cooked polyunsaturated fats, trans fats, saturated fats, foods high in free radicals, and foods that have oxidized.

10. A little of every natural food is helpful.

11. A diet high in vegetables and whole grains along with some fruit, animal foods, raw foods, and fermented foods, as well as one that is primarily made up of natural foods straight from the land, could be thought of as being helpful for human consumption.

12. This information could make a useful starting point for developing your own intuition for choosing food.

CHAPTER TWENTY-FOUR
Liquids

Macrobiotics, the large view (macro) of life (bios), has been the most significant gift I've received this lifetime. There is real meaning and joy in being able to help oneself, and then others, reclaim their health and happiness, whether over a shared meal, in a cooking class, at a speaking engagement, or in a nutrition counseling session. Over the last thirty-five years, many eating plans have come to light, but none measure up in terms of substance to the simple yet profound wisdom of macrobiotics. Science now confirms what macrobiotics has always represented, that a diet and lifestyle based on whole grains and vegetables, with smaller amounts of beans and soy foods, and even smaller amounts of fruits, nuts, seeds, and organic animal foods for those who want them, is the best way to heal both ourselves and our planet. Brilliant!

—MEREDITH MCCARTY, macrobiotic counselor, teacher, and cookbook author

Our bodies are mostly made up of water. About seventy percent of the human body is liquid. Maintaining the ideal fluid balance and hydrating our cells is vital for good health. We typically lose just over five pints (or about two and a half liters) of fluid in a typical day through urination and sweating; this needs to be replenished through drinking and absorbing the water in our food. Generally, a natural foods diet with a few cups of tea will contain more than five pints of water. In addition, drinking some good-quality water daily may aid the process of ridding our bodies of unwanted substances.

HOW MUCH

There is much discussion on how much water to drink. As we discussed in the "Listening to Our Bodies" section in Chapter Twenty-One, there are so many variables that it would be impossible to come up with a firm answer. The best we could say is that we require somewhere between nothing and five pints of drinking water, depending on how much water is in our food, the humidity in the air, how much we sweat, and to what extent we need to urinate to restore our sodium/potassium and acid/alkaline balances.

Ultimately, the best we can do is be aware of the color of our urine and how we feel. If our urine has a light color and we urinate four to eight times a day, then we are probably consuming a reasonable amount of water.

Water

As we are mostly water, we could think of the energy of the water in our bodies connecting quickly with the energy of water coming into our bodies. It can feel refreshing to drink some clean, healthy water every day.

Water and teas have a long tradition of being used for healing, and drinking water can form a part of a healthy routine. At the same time, too much water can also overwork our bodies and, in particular, our kidneys.

Herbal Teas

Herbal teas, or tisanes, are made from a variety of plants, grasses, barks, dried flowers, seeds, roots, fruits, or herbs. By mixing the nutrients into water, they become easy to digest and readily absorbable. Popular examples are, chamomile, ginger, lemon, nettle, fresh mint, and rosehip teas.

The warmth of a tea helps warm and relax our stomachs, which makes it easier for us to absorb and take in the qualities of the tea. The tea itself will have properties that may be healing for you at the time. Most herb teas are alkaline-forming, and will help reduce overacidity in the stomach as well as helping to bring the body into a more alkaline state.

The nutrients in a tea can further influence our health and be a part of our healing. They are thought to bring about subtle chemical changes to our blood and other body fluids. In addition, a cup of herbal tea can be a strong mood changer, helping us feel calmer and more relaxed.

Traditionally, tea has been used in Japan as part of the tea ceremony, where the tea is an important part of the meditation process. You can try feeling the effects of different teas by first finding a relaxed state through the breathing meditation, and then drinking the tea and being aware of how it feels inside you. To do this effectively, you'll need to avoid getting distracted by the taste and smell of the tea and just focus on where it seems to go. Some teas, such as peppermint, may feel like they spread up toward your head, while a tea such as chamomile drifts downward. Kukicha might feel as though it stays in your stomach. You may find that on different days the tea has different influences on you depending on your energetic state at the time.

Water Filters

Many people use water filters for purifying tap water piped into the home. Depending on the filter, these can take out chlorine, iron, pesticides, fluoride, lead, heavy metals, salts, and bacteria. This is particularly useful if you live in an area where the water quality is poor. However, one of the problems with a water filter is that it can take out too much. It's possible that consuming regular impurities, ideally organic impurities, exercises our immune system, making us less prone to serious illness in our stomachs or intestines. Another issue is that some filters make the water acidic; this can ultimately compromise our health, particularly when combined with an acid-forming diet.

Distilled Water

Distilled water is made by boiling water so it turns to steam, and then condensing it back to water. This purifies the water, leaving nothing but pure water. This can be unhealthy, in that we're used to taking in a range of minerals with our water; drinking distilled water could actually leach minerals and electrolytes out of our bodies with long-term use. In addition, distilled water can become acidic when it comes into contact with air, ultimately bringing us to a more acidic state if consumed regularly.

Bottled Water

Bottled waters often come from mountains or wells, and contain a variety of minerals and other substances dissolved from the ground. In theory, these can be very healthy; however, if they come in plastic bottles they may contain potentially harmful toxic substances that leach into the water from the plastic container.

If you're fortunate enough to live close to a source of healthy spring or well water, you could collect the water in glass or stainless steel containers to reduce contamination. When buying bottled water, try to get water in glass bottles.

Bottled water of any kind may have been stored for long periods, depending on where it comes from and how it is distributed. This may allow the water to stagnate in terms of its energy. Some bottled water is simply bottled public water, the same you would get from your own tap.

Tap Water

One of the advantages of tap water is that it is fresh if used regularly. Some impurities will evaporate if the water is left standing for an hour. Depending on where you live, tap water will have strict quality controls—but it may have chlorine and fluoride added to the water. Running water through lead piping also may compromise the quality of tap water.

Tap water could be argued to be environmentally better than bottled, as bottled water requires transportation and the manufacture of bottles, along with creating issues regarding waste.

WATER IN FOODS

Natural, fresh, unprocessed, whole, living foods tend to have a high water content. This is particularly true of vegetables and fruits. The plant has naturally filtered the water in these foods and, if the water has come from the ground, it will include various minerals from the land where the plant has grown. In this form, the water will be alkaline forming. So you could experiment and see to what extent you can satisfy most of your need for hydration from fruits and vegetables, and be aware of how this feels.

SURFACE TENSION

Water with a high surface tension will bead, whereas water with a low surface tension spreads out easily. In theory, the water with low surface tension will hydrate our cells more easily and be close to the low surface tension found in the fluids around our cells. It has been claimed that one of the reasons that the people of Hunza enjoying such longevity is that their water has a low surface tension.

Vinegars naturally contain acetic acid, which has the effect of reducing the surface tension of a liquid. You can try mixing a little apple cider vinegar with water to lower its surface tension and see if you feel better hydrated. Some people find that drinking water with a capful of apple cider vinegar reduces stress-related headaches. Using vinegars in our food can further help reduce the surface tension of liquids.

PH BALANCE

You can make water or tea more alkaline-forming by adding some lime or lemon juice. In addition, parsley, kudzu, *umeboshi,* and sea vegetables can be highly alkaline-forming. You could create your own special tea by mixing up any of these ingredients. For example, simmer kombu, a sea vegetable, for ten minutes, add a bunch of parsley, simmer a further ten minutes, take out the parsley and kombu, and squeeze in some lemon. You could also add a pinch of an *umeboshi* to your herbal tea or thicken a tea with a teaspoon of kudzu.

If you feel adventurous, experiment and be aware of how you feel to see if you can create your own ultimate alkalizing tea. Look in the recipe section for more ideas.

PRACTICAL EXERCISES

1. Adjust the amount of water and teas you drink so that your urine has a pale yellow color. Ignore the first urine of the day, as this is normally darker.
2. Try different herbal teas and note the effects they have on your body, energy, and emotions.
3. Try to go for month without drinking any water from plastic bottles.
4. Fill a cup with tap water and leave it out to stand for an hour. Drink it and see how you feel.

5. Try mixing a capful of apple cider vinegar into a glass of water. Drink it and be aware of its effect on you.

6. Make several herbal teas; sample one after the other and gain experience in feeling their effects on your body. Try meditating before each, and continue your meditation while sipping so you can feel where the energy of the tea goes in your body. See if you can describe the different qualities you feel as each tea enters your body.

SUMMARY

1. Water makes up about seventy percent of our bodies.
2. We need to replace about five pints of liquid per day.
3. We typically take in about five pints of fluid from a natural foods diet and two or three cups of tea.
4. As there are so many variables, it's impossible to say how much water a person should drink. The color of your urine is a sensible guide.
5. Water and teas have a long history of being used for healing.
6. Herb teas are warming, easy to digest, and quick to absorb, making them a helpful home remedy.
7. Calming teas can change our moods and can be a helpful influence on meditation.
8. You can feel the effect of drinking tea for yourself by getting into a meditative state and feeling the tea enter your body.
9. Water filters can be useful for taking out impurities, but they may take out useful substances and in some cases make the water acidic.
10. Distilled water is sterile and drinking it may lead to a loss of minerals and electrolytes over time.
11. Bottled water often comes from a healthy natural source, but it can be stored for long periods of time in plastic containers that add toxins to the water.
12. Ideally, use glass or stainless steel containers for storing water.
13. Tap water may contain impurities, but it's fresh and more ecologically sound than bottled water.

14. Water with a low surface tension my help us hydrate our cells more easily.

15. Adding vinegar to water or salads will slightly reduce the water tension.

16. We can make water or tea more alkaline-forming by adding lemon juice, lime juice, parsley, sea vegetables, *umeboshi,* or kudzu.

CHAPTER TWENTY-FIVE

Sleep

Macrobiotics is not a diet. Macrobiotics is an orderly approach to diet and lifestyle. Through principles of harmony, balance, and change, we continually learn how to make healthier choices in our eating habits, diet, activities, and lifestyles.

Macrobiotics is also based on the understanding that spiritual health, the development of endless appreciation for all of life, leads to mental, emotional, and physical health. The healthy choices we each make on a daily basis also benefit society and the environment.

—DENNY WAXMAN, macrobiotic counselor, founder of the
Strengthening Health Institute, and author of *The Great Life Diet*

Sleep has long been recognized as essential for good health. George Ohsawa included it as one of his seven essential ingredients for good health. Good sleep may play as big a role in cleansing our bodies of free radicals as eating foods high in antioxidants.

STAGES OF SLEEP

Stage One: Light Sleep

During the first stage of sleep, our muscle activity slows down and slight twitching may occur. This is a period of light sleep, and we can awaken easily.

Stage Two: True Sleep

Within ten minutes of light sleep, we enter stage two, which lasts around twenty minutes. Our breathing patterns and heart rates start to slow down. This period accounts for the largest portion of our sleep.

Stages Three and Four: Deep Sleep

During stage three, the brain begins to produce delta waves, a type of wave that is large and slow. Breathing and heart rate reach their lowest levels. Stage four is made up of rhythmic breathing and limited muscle activity.

Many of our cells show increased production and reduced breakdown of proteins during deep sleep. These proteins are the building blocks needed for cell growth, and for repair of damage from factors like stress and ultraviolet rays during the previous day. Children and young adults also release growth hormones during deep sleep.

Activity in the parts of our brains that control decision making, emotions, and social interactions are greatly reduced during deep sleep, suggesting that deep sleep helps us enjoy optimal emotional and social functioning the next day.

REM Sleep

The first rapid eye movement (REM) period usually begins about seventy to ninety minutes after we fall asleep. We typically experience three to five REM episodes a night.

During REM sleep, our brains are very active; this is the period when most dreams occur. Our eyes dart around, our breathing rate and blood pressure rise. However, our bodies are effectively sedated. After REM sleep, the whole cycle begins again.

REPAIR

The neurons that control our sleep interact with our immune systems. It's thought that good sleep helps our immune systems function fully, and that we're more prone to illness after a period of poor sleep, as our immune system becomes impaired. Many hormones that trigger or regulate various body functions are released during sleep or right before sleep. Growth hormones, for example, are released during sleep, vital to growing children but also for processes like muscle repair. There are a variety of associations with poor sleep and mental or emotional disorders. For example, people suffering from depression often wake in the early hours of the morning and cannot get back to sleep.

Our pineal glands produce melatonin during our deep sleep phases. Melatonin is a powerful antioxidant that also regulates our immune systems and is thought to inhibit the growth of cancer cells. Our production of melatonin can be disrupted by a lack of sleep or interrupted sleep. Light and the presence of alternating electromagnetic fields are both considered to decrease melatonin production. As we age, our pineal glands slowly calcify and reduce their production of melatonin. As we get older, it therefore becomes more important to sleep in a way that maximizes our production of melatonin.

DREAMS

Sigmund Freud, considered the father of psychoanalysis, believed that dreaming was a safety valve for unconscious desires. It may be that during the night we realign our energetic bodies and in the process throw off emotions. Our dreams may be the associated images that go with the departing emotions. Dreams can reflect our excess emotional energy, and a regular theme can be an indication of what kind of daytime thoughts and emotions are disturbing us.

Sometimes we can have what Michio Kushi calls a "true dream," where our dream appears profound and insightful, and as if it contains a special message for us. These dreams may come through a connection to the energy of our universe; perhaps we are only able to receive this energy when we are in a particular relaxed state.

INTUITION AND SUBCONSCIOUS

During the night, our intuition and subconscious continue to work; without the distraction of running our active bodies and minds, we can dedicate more attention to other issues. For this reason, you may find it helps to consider any problems you are seeking an answer to before you go to sleep. This may allow you to continue seeking a solution while asleep. You might find an interesting answer pops into your head when you wake. In my experience, it works best if I run through the issue a few times in my head as I go to sleep.

It helps to keep some paper and a pen next to your bed just in case you wake with a wonderful new insight or revelation. If nothing happens after the first night, persevere for a few nights. Before going to sleep, try getting yourself into a warm, content state where you feel complete. Then, imagine feeling ready to move on and leave your body. Ask yourself the question, What I would have to do between now and the end of my life to feel I can pass on without any regrets? See if anything pops into your head when you wake up.

CAFFEINE

Caffeine in coffee, chocolate, and some soft drinks can, for some, interfere with our sleep. This may compromise our health and lead to poor alertness the following day, prompting the desire for more caffeine. If you want to drink coffee, it would make sense to drink it during the morning to give your body the maximum amount of time to get rid of the caffeine before you sleep.

SUGGESTIONS FOR GOOD SLEEP

What would help us enjoy a healthy night's sleep and prepare us for the next day?

To make the most of our melatonin production, it would help to be in a deep sleep between the hours of 12 a.m. and 3 a.m. This would mean going to bed at 11 p.m. to allow time to fall asleep and get to the deep sleep part of our sleeping cycles.

As alternating electromagnetic fields can inhibit the production of melatonin, it is helpful to ensure you are not sleeping in these fields. Keep all plugged-in electrical items well away from your bed. This would include radios, alarm clocks, televisions, computers, DVD players, night-lights, cell phones, hands-free phone base stations, and answering machines. I would suggest you keep any electrical equipment at least one yard or meter from your bed. It would be general good practice to keep your bedroom as free from electrical equipment as possible. Battery-operated clocks do not create a harmful field.

Synthetic materials create electrostatic fields, and these can interfere with the electrical signals running through our bodies. This can disturb the electrical impulses flowing between our hearts, minds, and bodies. It's possible that any disturbance will impair our ability to heal our energetic bodies and release emotions. Examples of materials that could be made from synthetic fibers and affect your sleep are carpets, sheets, mattresses, duvets, blankets, pillows, and pajamas. I would suggest using pure cotton sheets, pajamas, duvet covers, and pillow covers. Pure wool carpets and blankets would be ideal. Finding mattresses made from natural fibers can be more of a challenge. In my home we use a pure cotton futon; you could also look for a mattress made from layers of horsehair, wool, and cotton. Try natural feathers or silk for the filling for duvets and pillows. A wooden bed frame will be neutral and not upset the earth's magnetic field around you.

In feng shui thinking, it helps to create a relaxing, comfortable atmosphere for good sleep. Try to fill your bedroom with soft surfaces. Carpets, rugs, long curtains, big cushions, and bedding can all make a room feel more soft and secure for good sleep. Reduce hard, sharp surfaces such as sharp edges, large mirrors, or stone flooring to create a warmer feel. Think about colors that will be calming and help you drop into a peaceful mood before falling asleep.

To improve your melatonin production, make sure your bedroom is dark at night. Use blackout curtains if necessary and avoid sleeping in the glow of night-lights, candles, or electrical equipment.

You may find that you sleep better in a certain area of your room, or even with the top of your head pointing in a certain direction. Many herding animals naturally sleep so that their spine is aligned with the earth's magnetic field. This means they sleep north to south. This would suggest sleeping with the top of our head pointing north or south. There is some speculation that we then interact with the earth's magnetic field in a way that promotes better sleep and healing over the night. However, you might find through your own experimentation that another direction suits you better; it makes sense to set up your bedroom in whatever way creates the best sleeping environment for you.

Generally, eating about three hours before you go to sleep will help you sleep well and allow your body to go through its healing cycles without the distraction of trying to simultaneously digest and absorb food. Similarly, it would make sense to adjust your drinking habits so that you don't have to get up during the night to urinate, as this disturbs your deep sleep and delta sleep parts of your sleeping cycle.

PRACTICAL EXERCISES

1. Before you go to sleep, try your breathing meditation and consider any issues you are concerned about to see if you have any insight in the morning.
2. Try not drinking coffee, eating chocolate, or consuming other caffeine-rich foods for a month; be aware of how you sleep.
3. Experiment by going to sleep at 11 p.m. every night for a week and be aware of your health during the day.
4. Move any electrical equipment so it's at least one yard or meter from your bed. Assess your quality of sleep and general health after a month.
5. Try to use pure cotton for your bedding and other natural materials for duvets and mattresses. Be aware of your sleep and health over the next month.
6. Make sure your bedroom is dark at night. Review your sleep and health after a month.
7. Try to eat no less than three hours before you go to sleep for a week and be aware of how you feel in the morning.

SUMMARY

1. Good sleep is essential for good health.
2. Sleep consists of cycles; part of the cycle includes a period of deep sleep when we repair cells.
3. Our pineal glands produce melatonin, which is a powerful antioxidant used for repairing our DNA.
4. Our production of melatonin can be disrupted by light and alternating EMFs from electrical equipment.

5. Dreams may come from our bodies throwing off spent energy and emotions.

6. During the night, the subconscious can process issues and provide solutions for us in the morning.

7. In some people, caffeine interferes with deep sleep and upsets the cycle.

8. Being in a deep sleep between 12 a.m. and 3 a.m. aids the production of melatonin.

9. Synthetic materials, such nylon, create a static charge of electricity; this may interfere with our natural electrical impulses.

10. A soft, cozy, comfortable bedroom may help create the ideal atmosphere for sleep.

11. You could experiment with moving your bed to different places in a the bedroom to see if a certain position works best for deep sleep.

12. Eating early and restricting the amount of liquid you consume before sleep may help you get a full, uninterrupted night's sleep.

CHAPTER TWENTY-SIX

Skin Care

Macrobiotics initially provided a refreshing well of hope for me, and, over time, has provided constructive tools for me to live a better and more satisfying life. When a doctor informed me that I had a latex allergy and food-related cross reactions that had "no cure," I despaired. Learning about and practicing a whole foods diet based on macrobiotic principles has dramatically improved my quality of life in aspects that I had never imagined were related to the food I was eating. Health and wellness are definitely holistic! Imagine my surprise when healing my allergies also meant healing my fear of public speaking.

—LESLIE ASHBURN, macrobiotic teacher and personal chef

The skin is the human body's biggest organ; it plays an important role in eliminating different waste substances. It forms a partially porous barrier between our bodily fluids and the environment around us. In addition, our skin is important to us, as it reflects our appearance; we often place great value on having what we consider to be healthy-looking skin.

Healthy skin breaths easily, is flexible, and allows fluids to pass through small openings called pores. If you sweat all over your body when hot, your skin is probably breathing well. You can test the flexibility of your skin by pulling the skin on the back of your hand and seeing how long it takes to return to its natural state.

Good blood circulation can improve the condition of our skin and slow the process of aging, as well as encourage our natural oils to come through to the surface of our skin. We are aware of our skin through the nerves that enable us to feel through it. The sensation of being touched can provide great pleasure, affecting our moods and energy bodies.

Our skin also protects us from ultraviolet radiation from the sun. Too great and too long an exposure to UV radiation burns and damages the DNA of our skin.

BREATHING

To be able to breathe well, our skin needs to be open and free from blockages. Sometimes our skin's ability to breathe can be impaired by having too much fat below the surface. Too much fat can slow the flow of blood and liquids to the surface. In addition, putting creams on our skin can clog up our pores from the outside. Over time, using creams on our body can, in some people, reduce the ability to release waste through the skin.

Deodorants that block the sweat glands interfere with our natural elimination of waste. It would make more sense to use deodorants that allow us to sweat but alter any unpleasant smells. Another alternative would be to simply wash more often throughout the day.

SKIN RUBBING

One way to improve the blood flow to our skin is to rub it. Try rubbing your body with a hot, damp cloth. Simply dip a cotton flannel or small hand towel in hot water, wring it out, and fold it into a pad that you can hold easily. Then, rub your bare skin with the cloth. Once it cools, put the cloth back into the hot water, wring it out, and continue. Spend more time on parts of your body that do not turn red as easily as other areas.

I would not recommend rubbing the face, as most facial muscles are connected to bones only at one end; over-rubbing can elongate these muscles, leading to looser cheeks.

Natural skin care and beauty expert Dr. Hauschka suggests that rubbing and aggressive cleansers actually harm our facial skin. He recommends simply pressing and rolling a warm damp cloth onto our skin to gently remove dirt, oil, and makeup without disturbing the skin's natural balance of water and oil on its surface.

FACE CARE

One of the challenges is to remove dirt, makeup, and waste from the surface of our faces without damaging them in the process. Some of the dirt can be abrasive and, if agitated, damage the surrounding skin.

The surfaces of our skin have what is called an acid mantle. The acid mantle is a very fine, slightly acidic film on the surface of the skin that acts as a barrier to bacteria, viruses, and other potential contaminants that might penetrate the skin. These contaminants and other chemicals are primarily alkaline in nature, and the skin's moderate acidity helps to neutralize their chemical effects.

Soaps, scrubs, and exfoliants can strip our faces of natural protection, in some people risking dryness, irritated skin, and premature aging. The idea of Dr. Hauschka's gentle press and roll with a warm face cloth is that we can carefully remove excess dirt while leaving our protective acid mantle intact. In addition, this method stimulates the flow of lymphatic fluids under the skin of our faces.

SOAPS

Soaps can affect the delicate ecosystem that is present on the surface of our skin. You may find it helps to use natural soaps that are mild, and to use them sparingly on the parts of your body that you most need to clean.

MOISTURIZERS

Anita Roddick, founder of The Body Shop, once famously claimed that moisturizers to be the only cosmetics of any worth. The aim of moisturizers is to prevent the skin from drying out, and to help protect it from some airborne pollution. As our skin repairs overnight, it would make sense to use a moisturizer during the day and leave our skin free to breathe during the night.

OILS

There has been a long history of using oils on our skin. Greeks and Romans traditionally used olive oils to keep their skin moist during the summer. You may feel that applying oil to your skin helps it remain elastic. Many women have found regular use of oil on their skin during pregnancy has helped their skin return to its natural condition after giving birth. We can also use oils for massage; typically, almond oil is a good base oil. We can mix this with other oils to create the aroma and feel that suits us best.

SUN

The sun is helpful for helping us synthesize vitamin D. Exposure to sunshine can help open the skin and allow waste to come up to the surface. At the same time, our skin can be harmed by excessive exposure to ultraviolet radiation from the sun. Fair-skinned people are most at risk, as there's less melanin present. In addition, our skin can become more sensitive as we age. In medical terms, sunburn can permanently damage the DNA of our skin, making us more sensitive to the sun.

If you're concerned about exposure to the sun, it would make sense to avoid sunshine during the middle of the day and only expose yourself to sunshine in the early morning or late afternoon.

FEET

Over time, we can experience a buildup of dry skin on our feet, which develops into calluses. This thick dry skin reduces the flow of blood and energy to the surface of the skin and increases the risk of stagnation. To free up the energy in and around our feet, it would help to remove calluses by rubbing them gently with a pumice stone.

PERFUMES

Try a variety of naturally scented perfumes until you find the smell that feels good to you. Remember that perfumes are liquid, and they will be absorbed into your skin and can affect your blood.

Strong perfumes can alter your ability to experience other natural smells around you, reducing your connection to nature and your environment. This can affect your relationship with your food, as the smell of your food is an important part of your enjoyment of a meal.

LOVE

Whenever you wash, massage, scrub, dry, or apply lotions, try to do so with love and gentleness. Treat yourself kindly, and use the time you are in contact with your skin to express the natural love you have for yourself. Practice being tender and gentle with yourself: you are special and someone to be cherished. Imagine you are holding a baby, and perform each touch with care and a natural affection.

PRACTICAL EXERCISES

1. Try not using deodorants for two days and see if you really need them. Stopping coffee, garlic, strong spices, cheese, and meat at the same time can help, as they sometimes alter our body odors.
2. Experiment with not using creams for a week to discover whether they are necessary for your skin.
3. Rub the skin on your body every day for a week with a hot, damp cloth, and be aware of any changes to your circulation.
4. Gently press and roll a warm cotton cloth over your face to cleanse for a month, and be aware of any changes to the appearance of the skin on your face.
5. Use mild soaps or cleansing creams sparingly for a month, and observe any changes to the appearance of your skin.
6. For a month, try gently washing your skin before bed and leaving it free from any creams or oils so it can breath overnight; be aware of any changes in the quality of your skin.
7. If you're close to someone, try giving each other a gentle massage once a week and, if you like, massage a natural oil into each other's skin.
8. Use a pumice stone to remove excess dry skin from your feet, and be aware of how you feel.

9. If you like to wear perfumes, experiment with a variety of natural perfumes to find the scent that suits you best, while allowing you to experience the natural smells around you.

10. When you touch your skin, do so with love, care, tenderness, and gentleness.

SUMMARY

1. Our skin is the biggest and heaviest organ we have.

2. We breathe through the pores in our skin and use this process to eliminate waste.

3. Excess creams, oils, and lotions can block the pores, impairing the skin's ability to breathe.

4. Deodorants can upset the skin's natural ability to breathe and eliminate waste.

5. Gently massaging and rubbing the skin can help blood circulation.

6. Gently pressing and rolling a warm, damp cotton cloth across your face can remove dirt, oils, and makeup without harming the skin.

7. The surface of our faces has an acid mantle that protects the skin. It's helpful to keep this layer intact rather than harm it with soaps, scrubs, or exfoliants.

8. Soaps can upset the delicate ecosystem of the skin surface.

9. To allow your skin to best repair and regenerate itself overnight, you can try leaving it bare.

10. Excessive exposure to sunlight can damage the skin and harm its DNA.

11. A buildup of dry skin on our feet can reduce blood circulation and increase the risk of energy stagnation.

12. Perfumes can overwhelm our sensitivity to other smells and disconnect us from our food and environment.

13. Whatever we put on our skin can find its way into our bodies and bloodstreams.

14. Every time we touch our skin, we have the opportunity to express a love of ourselves.

CHAPTER TWENTY-SEVEN
Exercise and Stretching

One of the most important things that happened in my life has been to be introduced to a great way of life that has been named "macrobiotics." I remember the first lectures and seminars that I attended on the subject: They made so much sense that I didn't feel like asking any questions. Everything completely met my needs of the moment; of course, I had plenty of questions soon after. I also remember having an almost naive pleasure on discovering new foods, some of which were really quite strange to me.

As I started reducing many of the foods I used to eat, I realized that I could now make more sensible and wise choices. It was a beautiful period of my life. Then, there was living and sharing this lifestyle with my husband and my children. It has been a wonderful journey toward finding a meaning to everything that unfolds—sometimes easy, other times more challenging.

Today I rejoice for all the steps walked in this great life; they made me much more aware and, above all, more authentic, truthful, and coherent. It is good to take care of myself and others as well as the environment that surrounds us. It is good to feel an enormous respect and love toward the magnificence of this universe. It is good to contribute, doing the best I can.

It is good to be here.

—EUGENIA VARATOJO, macrobiotic cooking teacher,
author, cook, and director of the Macrobiotic Institute of Portugal

If we think of our bodies as energy systems, we have energy coming in, in the form of calories from food and oxygen from the air, and some of this energy then is used up by physically moving our bodies around.

How we use up this energy can be as influential on our health as how we get it. Our exercise and stretching regimes have an influence on our blood circulation, blood pressure, weight, muscles, hearts, skin, bones, lungs, and nervous systems.

EXERCISE

There are many forms of exercise. Gardening, cleaning, walking, and other similar activities require movement and use up energy. These form a gentle approach to exercise that involve movement and rest. We can sustain this kind of activity for most of the day.

Aerobic exercise is when we exercise at a rate that elevates our pulse and requires faster breathing. Here our body is expending energy more rapidly, but not so quickly that we could not, for example, hold a conversation with someone. This could be achieved through activities like fast walking, jogging, running, tennis, football, basketball, swimming, and volleyball.

Anaerobic exercise takes us to a point where, through intense, vigorous exercise, we create more lactic acid than we can eliminate from our blood. This is generally not recommended; for most people it is not particularly healthy. Examples would be running up a mountain, running up a hill carrying a heavy weight, lifting very heavy weights quickly, or fighting.

Aerobic exercise causes our hearts to pump our blood more rapidly so that we can move energy to our muscles more quickly. This strengthens our hearts and improves our blood circulation as the blood moves freely though our arteries to all our muscles. At the same time we will experience an increased rate of breathing, as we need to absorb more oxygen. This enriches our blood with oxygen. In the process, we exercise our lungs and increase in the rate of biological processes that get oxygen into our blood.

Our bodies respond well to use. By using our muscles regularly, we keep them in a state of good health. Too little use and they waste away. Similarly, being physically active keeps our nervous systems exercised and healthy. Research indicates that regular exercise even helps keep our bones healthy and reduces the risk of osteoporosis, a state where our bones lose mass and become brittle.

If you are exercising to lose weight, you'll need to exercise for long enough to use all the energy stored in your blood and muscles, so that you then start to convert fat back into energy. You may find the first twenty minutes or so of exercise is simply using available energy, and it is only after that, that you burn off energy reserves in the form of fat. Be careful not to simply generate a huge appetite through exercise, and then find that you eat the very foods that put weight back on. Try to organize yourself so that you'll be able to eat a healthy meal after exercising—in particular, a meal that won't raise your blood sugar quickly.

One of the great benefits of regular exercise is that we burn off calories and, unless we are trying to lose excess fat, require more calories to replace them. When we consume these extra calories, we have the opportunity to absorb many other useful nutrients with them if we eat healthy, natural foods. For example, eating an apple after exercising will bring in many useful vitamins, antioxidants, and phytonutrients (eating sugary cookies will replace the calories, but with fewer of the other potentially helpful nutrients). So we could say that regular exercise creates the demand for foods that will bring more healing nutrients to our body.

If you like to work out in a gym, bet aware of the difference between building up muscle mass, which is done by lifting heavy weights, and aerobic exercise, which can be experienced by moving lighter weights many times over a long duration. For example, running in place while lifting light weights in your hands can be an invigorating aerobic exercise. To build up muscles, it's recommended that you isolate a group of muscles and work them continuously. The risks of this approach are that you may develop your body in an unbalanced way and that you can injure your muscles through repetitive action. I find it better to go swimming or play a sport, as I naturally develop my body with a fuller range of movements. When I go to the gym, I use free weights rather than any machines in an attempt to use a greater variety of muscles.

You can also use certain types of more energetic yoga, tai chi, qi gong, and dance to develop your physical health.

Remember to do any kind of exercise with awareness. If you don't feel good during or after the exercise, it may not be the right exercise for you. Be aware of your physical, mental, and emotional state before and after exercising, so you can feel for yourself what kind of exercise works for you and how best to do it.

Interestingly, I find that when I feel tired and am about to end my exercise session, I can extend my stamina by going into my breathing meditation.

STRETCHING

As we age, we tend to lose our natural elasticity. Parts of our bodies become stiff, hard, rigid, and brittle. This can affect our muscles, bones, and joints. If this includes our blood vessels, then there's a risk of increased blood pressure.

Regular stretching helps us maintain our natural elasticity. You can stretch at any time and for as long as suits you. Generally, I recommend you start with long, slow stretches. Try to really feel the stretch. You may find that small adjustments make the stretch feel very different. For example, if you stretch your head to one side, turning your head slightly or moving it back or forward a little changes the stretch. With subtle adjustments, you can get the stretch so that it feels like you are elongating your stiff muscles.

Stretching works well with exercise, as when we exercise there is the risk that the muscles we work become slightly shorter. The muscles can retain lactic acid, and the muscle fibers may not always return to their optimum position. Stretching the muscles after exercise helps bring them back to their ideal state. Stretching before exercise can reduce the risk of injury. The older we get, the more we might need to stretch to complement our exercising.

You can create your own stretches by being aware of the parts of your body you want to stretch, and then finding a position that stretches out that part. Common stretches are touching your toes, bending to the side, kneeling and leaning backwards, twisting your back, sitting with your legs out straight and apart as far as possible and leaning forward, hanging off a bar, and joining your hands behind your upper back.

We can use stretching to help become more aware of our bodies. It's interesting to be aware of how we feel physically, mentally and emotionally after stretching. In theory, each time we stretch, we move our energetic bodies into a new shape; this change in energy will have a subtle influence on our minds and emotions.

PRACTICAL EXERCISES

1. Try going for a walk every day for ten days and see how you feel. You can walk to work, get off the bus early on your way to work, or just go out and walk to a park.

2. Experiment with taking on some kind of aerobic exercise at least twice a week. See if you can exercise continuously for more then twenty minutes. Be aware of how you feel after each session, and try different kinds of exercise until you find something you enjoy and that feels healthy.

3. Take up some form of physical activity, whether a hobby, sport, or other activity, and make the time to enjoy it at least once a week.

4. If you want to lose weight, try some form of aerobic exercise for more than thirty minutes every other day for a month. You may feel hungry after the exercise; it will help to have healthy food ready so you don't reach out for something that could put the weight back on.

5. If you like to work out at the gym, try using lighter free weights with more repetitions. See if you can add more variety to your routine so you work a bigger range of muscles.

6. Experiment with stretching for ten minutes before and after exercising.

7. Try ten minutes of stretching every day for a month and see if you become more flexible; be aware of how you feel after stretching.

8. If you have high blood pressure, try stretching and meditating on your breathing for ten minutes three times a day; after a month, have your blood pressure checked again.

SUMMARY

1. In addition to how we bring energy into our bodies through food and breathing, we can change our health through how we use some of that energy in the form of exercise.

2. Exercise can be a physical activity, sports, or aerobic exercise.

3. Regular exercise can help blood circulation and the health of our hearts, bones, nervous systems, muscles, and lungs.

4. Regular exercise can also play a part in maintaining our ideal weight, and in losing weight.

5. Exercise can increase our appetites, and there is a risk that we then eat the kinds of food that put weight back on.

6. A variety of exercise is likely to be most healthy.

7. If you go to a gym, try working with lighter weights and introducing more repetitions; be aware of the way you feel.

8. As we age, we tend to become more stiff, hard, rigid, and brittle.

9. Regular stretching can help us maintain our elasticity.

10. Start with long, slow stretches, and develop your own stretching routine by feeling the stretches and creating stretches that stretch the parts of your body that feel stiff.

11. Stretching before and after exercising can reduce the risk of injury and help prevent stiffness.

12. Try to exercise and stretch in a state of awareness, so you can find the kind of exercise or the stretches that are best for you.

CHAPTER TWENTY-EIGHT
Chanting

A postwar babe in the 1970s imagining a new paradigm: a sustainable, peaceful world! We lived simply, rode bikes to save fuel, marched against nuclear power, made bread, grew veggies, and knew that food nourished body and soul. Genetic modification was reported on the radio and people were being turned into consumers.

Michio and Aveline lectured in London on macrobiotics, explaining how all life in the universe is connected on a vibrational level between and beyond heaven and earth. They described the system of biological and spiritual evolution according to yin and yang tendencies and universal principles. This resonated deeply with my sense of the world, justice, and what it is to be a free, conscious human being.

Awesome, gracious, and practical, it brought me back to life. I have followed this path for thirty fascinating years and look forward to the next thirty.

I am truly thankful!

—R. ANNA MACKENZIE, cooking teacher and interior alignment counselor

SOUNDS

Any sound creates vibration. We hear sounds because the source of a sound vibrates the air, and that vibration stimulates tympanic membranes in our ears, which sends signals to our brains. Some sounds can be so intense that they vibrate our bones.

Sound is also useful for its ability to vibrate larger bones. This phenomenon means we can massage the inside of our bodies in a way that we cannot do with our hands. As the bones vibrate, they shake up the surrounding tissue and help move our blood. This also frees up our energetic bodies, encouraging stagnant energy to move while spreading constrained and intense energy. For this reason, many people use sound to help change their emotional states and physical conditions.

The Healing Power of Sound

In theory, any sound can have a healing component if it feels healing to you. Music, singing, oratory, chanting, or playing an instrument can all in some way use sound vibration to change our physical and emotional states. To make a significant difference to our physical bodies, the sound would need to be strong enough for us to feel the vibration in our bones. Chanting or singing can best do this.

It may be that this sonic vibration resonates with certain parts of our bodies, stimulating the energy there. This may be one reason why music can have such a powerful influence over our emotions.

Chanting

To chant, find a position where you feel comfortable. This could be standing, sitting, kneeling, or lying on your back. Start by breathing in fully and making a loud "ahh" sound. As you do this, be aware of which bones you feel vibrate. You might find that the lower the pitch, the lower in your body you feel the vibration. You can play with the sound and feel the difference.

Next, try making a long, loud "ooo" sound, and be aware of where you feel the vibration. This time, you may find it moves up your body to the area around your upper chest, throat, or jaw. Again, you can play with the pitch to feel how the vibration moves to different parts of your body.

Finally, try making an "mmm" sound, and again feel which bones vibrate. You may find this vibrates various bones in your throat and face, depending on the pitch. Play with making a high-pitched "mmm" sound and feel how high up in your head you can get the bones to vibrate.

You can then repeatedly make these sounds to vibrate different parts of your body in whatever way you feel would help you most. Alternatively, you can put all three sounds into one breath. You can start making an "ahh" sound, move to an "ooo" sound, and finish the long exhalation with an "mmm" sound. As you do this, you may feel the focus of vibration move up through from your ribs to your face. Try doing this three to six times, and be aware of how you feel. You could also try making the sounds in the reverse order by chanting "mmm, ooo, ahh" in one long breath, repeating for several breaths, and being aware of how you feel.

Singing

Singing essentially has the same influence as chanting, except that you are less able to hold a particular sound for an extended period of time to focus the vibration on a particular part of your body.

Singing a song with a range of notes will spread the sonic vibration over a wider range of bones and different parts of your body. Holding a note will focus the vibration more intensely on one part of your body.

The lyrics and melody of a song may in itself change your emotions and therefore your energy. Singing happy songs with a light tune might lift your mood and inspire you to feel more joyful. Singing with other people can have the effect of creating an energetic harmony, as each person tunes into creating and receiving sonic vibrations that are in harmony with the others.

Listening to Music

Although listening to music does not vibrate our bones in the same way that singing or chanting does, music does bathe us in sonic vibrations that subtly massage the exterior of our skin and influences our outer energy fields.

Some songs and melodies can excite and stimulate our peripheral energy fields, while others relax and soothe it. You may find there are pieces of music that help calm you so that you can more quickly get into your breathing meditation and go from your head to your heart.

There may be songs that you have formed positive associations with, such as a summer hit or a song you listened to frequently during happy times. It can be helpful to be aware of these, and see if you are simply listening to something for the associations or because it has a certain influence on your energetic body.

PRACTICAL EXERCISES

1. Try chanting "ahh," "ooo," and "mmm" sounds for three minutes each day for one month; reflect on how you feel.
2. Experiment with singing for a few minutes every day, and be aware of any changes in your mood.
3. Consider joining a choir or singing group, or having singing lessons, so you can sing with other people.
4. Be aware of the effect different types of music have on your emotional energy.

SUMMARY

1. Sounds create vibrations in the air that stimulate our ears, subtly massage our skin, and alter the outer part of our energetic bodies.
2. Chanting, singing, or talking can also vibrate bones in our bodies that massage the surrounding tissue.
3. Vibrating our bones through sound stimulates the blood flow around the bones.
4. Sonic vibration can influence our energetic bodies, helping us reach certain emotional states.
5. We can chant different sounds and vibrate different parts of our bodies.
6. Generally, the higher the pitch the more we vibrate bones that are higher in the body.
7. Singing sends a range of vibrational tones into our bodies, stirring up the energy in different places and vibrating different bones.
8. Singing can help us share certain harmonies of vibrational energy with other people in a group.
9. Music can help change our moods and energies.
10. We can form emotional associations with certain songs; listening to those songs again can help re-create past emotions.

CHAPTER TWENTY-NINE
Natural Immunity

Many people use macrobiotics to improve health. I overcame allergies by switching from a dairy-and-fruit diet to a whole-grain-and-fresh-vegetables one. What moved me the most in George Ohsawa's writing, however, was his call to give back to macrobiotics. As I gave back, I received more. Macrobiotics is much more than a diet—it is a set of universal principles that help us recognize our connection to the Infinite Source (Oneness) of all beings and things. With this awareness, we replace our separating thoughts of sickness, unhappiness, and conflict with the unifying truth of unconditional love.

—CARL FERRÉ, president of the George Ohsawa Macrobiotic Foundation, author of the *Pocket Guide to Macrobiotics*, and teacher and organizer of French Meadows Summer Camp

Our immune systems are our biological internal healing systems. This is where our bodies perform incredible feats to be aware of potential dangers and to protect us and keep us in good health. The health of our immune system is instrumental in keeping us in good health and for longevity.

Our immune systems recognize when we have been exposed to a potentially harmful substance, and then react by creating a situation where the substance cannot survive. To help our immune systems react quickly, they have memories of previous incidents so that they can repeat their previous successful strategies.

Areas where we are most regularly exposed to exterior elements are our noses, sinuses, mouths, throats, stomachs, intestines, and lungs. Here our immune systems are active on a regular basis.

Problems can occur when our immune systems are weak or less reactive, leaving us vulnerable to infectious illnesses. With some health issues, such as allergies, arthritis, and diabetes, the immune system appears to overreact and even harm our own healthy cells. Our immune systems are also responsible for detecting cancer cells and moving them out of the body.

One theory is that if we exercise our immune systems on a regular basis, they simply becomes stronger and increase their memories of potential harmful substances and how to deal with them effectively. Through regular use from childhood, the immune system is better able to differentiate between real threats and imagined threats. It may be that allergies partially come about due to a lack of practice.

This would suggest not to be obsessive about living in an overly clean environment, including our drinking water and food. Eating root and ground vegetables with their skins will introduce some earth to our intestines. This will be more effective if we don't wash the vegetables too thoroughly. Simply brushing soil off vegetables from the garden and giving them a brief rinse will leave particles of dirt on the skins. Similarly, vegetables and fruits that are eaten raw will still have some natural organic matter on their surfaces that can gently exercise our immune systems.

Exposing ourselves to small amounts of organic dirt regularly could help form efficient immune systems. Living in a clean environment with washed foods and sterile water risks leaving us more vulnerable to outside substances and having a reduced capacity to deal with infections and viruses. This could mean a bout of food poisoning has a greater and more harmful effect on someone who has not regularly tested his or her immune system through the regular consumption of impurities.

Even scratches and small cuts can help us maintain efficient immune systems. An activity like gardening exposes us to dirt, scratches, and cuts that combine to strengthen our immune systems. It's even better if we eat the occasional fruit or vegetable straight from our garden while working with them.

Vegetables and fruits tend to be high in the minerals, vitamins, and phytonutrients that best help our immune systems function well. In addition, they can be grouped into the category of being alkaline-forming foods. There is speculation that a more alkaline internal body environment favors our immune systems.

In addition, there is some suggestion that stress can decrease the effectiveness of our immune systems, while positive thinking can increase their effectiveness. Practices like meditating on our breathing and feeling a love for ourselves may boost our immune systems.

From the research currently available, it would seem that a diet high in vegetables, fruits, and raw foods will further increase the effectiveness of our nervous systems. In the end, it is up to us to be aware of how effectively our immune systems operate; this can be measured by how often we become ill.

PRACTICAL EXERCISES

1. Try eating fruits and vegetables with the skins on for three months, and see if you prefer them.
2. Increase your consumption of vegetables, fruits, and fresh, raw foods for six months and be aware of any changes in your immune system.
3. Try not to be obsessed with cleanliness; expose yourself to some dirt on a regular basis for a month and be aware of whether you feel more resistant to infections.
4. Get involved in gardening or working with the soil for a month and be aware of how you feel.
5. Use regular breathing meditations to relax and avoid stress. Note the effect on your immune system.

SUMMARY

1. Our immune systems recognize threats to our health and protect us from those threats.
2. Our lungs and digestive systems are common places where our immune systems need to be active.
3. If our immune systems are not working properly, we can be susceptible to infectious illness, allergies, arthritis, and cancer.
4. Our immune systems build up memories, recognizing sources of potential harm and the best way to protect us.

5. Dirt, scratches, small cuts, impurities in food, and airborne viruses can all exercise our immune systems and add to their memories of how to keep us healthy.

6. Stress may reduce the effectiveness of our immune systems, while positive thinking and meditation may increase their effectiveness.

7. Diets high in vegetables, fruits, and raw foods can provide the nutrients required for our immune systems to work to their full potential. If there is some organic dirt on the skin of these foods, it will further exercise our immune systems.

PART FIVE

MACROBIOTIC PRINCIPLES

There are various macrobiotic principles we can draw on to help us ask questions of the world we live in and gain new and different insights into ourselves and, in particular, our relationships to food and other external influences.

Here we will explore the macrobiotic principle of change, see how this can affect our own thinking, and see how it has changed our interpretations of macrobiotics over the years.

We will look at Dr. Christoph Wilhelm Hufeland's and traditional Chinese views of living energy and how this can give us a different way of thinking about food. Sagen Ishizuka, George Ohsawa, and Herman Aihara placed an emphasis on acid and alkaline in using food to help recover our health; I will describe how we can test ourselves and what foods are acid- or alkaline-forming.

We will also look at the glycemic index and load, which has no history in macrobiotic practice but can provide useful information in terms of which foods raise our blood sugar more quickly.

Yin and yang have been a huge part of Chinese philosophy and medicine, and George Ohsawa introduced them to his version of macrobiotics. He described yin and yang as looking at the world through magical spectacles.

There is a wealth of Chinese history dedicated to the five elements, and these principles can be interesting when looking at food and health. Michio and Aveline Kushi taught and wrote about the five elements and how we can use them in our understanding of food.

By studying a little of the history of macrobiotics, we can appreciate its evolution over the last two thousand years and use all aspects of it. This helps us be more flexible in our practices and draw on a broader range of people's ideas and experience.

CHAPTER THIRTY
Change

One thing that everyone from scientists to philosophers to macrobiotic thinkers agree on is that our only constant is change. The world as we know it appears to be continually changing, whether it's the expansion of our galaxy or changes in the weather. Every day we change. We age slightly, perhaps feel healthier, learn from the previous day, and evolve based on our experience. Some people change more than others, but it's hard to be immune from the process of change.

Change tends to make nonsense of fixed ideas, dogma, rigid thinking, and set rules. What works today may not work the same way tomorrow. Time ensures that we cannot stand still, and part of the macrobiotic philosophy that George Ohsawa imparted was that embracing change is part of our life's journey. This is a common theme in Taoism and Zen Buddhism. It has also become a profound theme in scientific thinking.

Sometimes we experience huge shifts in our common understanding of the universe, and these are called paradigm shifts. Examples of this would be going from thinking that our planet was flat to thinking it is spherical, or going from thinking we were the center of our solar system to thinking we are orbiting the sun. There have been many such changes in scientific, religious, and new age thinking; this leads me to ask the question, Was it worth anyone clinging to any belief at the time? If our current beliefs are destined to be replaced by something else, is it really worth spending time feeling stressed if our beliefs are challenged? Do we need to prove ourselves right if the issue we are arguing over will one day be obsolete anyway? Have we simply adopted and used beliefs to define us, and in doing so become distracted from our true selves? Is this why we get so attached to our beliefs?

One way of thinking about change is to consider that if we don't change, we inevitably get left behind by a changing world and the changing perception of our world. In effect, we lose harmony with everything around us.

This is most relevant to people who live by ideas, concepts, or rules. Take something like nutritional science—anyone reviewing its evolution over the last sixty years will be amazed at how many changes there have been in our understanding of nutrition, and by how much nutritional advice has swung from glorifying one set of foods to another.

During the 1950s and '60s, meat, eggs, and dairy foods were the champions of healthy eating; then, in the '70s, fruits and vegetables became the ideal healthy foods. By the '80s, the saturated fat in meat, eggs, and dairy foods was claimed to be the main cause of heart disease and margarine or vegetable oils the savior. By the late '90s it became apparent that margarine, hydrogenated oils, and polyunsaturated fats in cooking could be doing just as much harm, contributing to rising rates of cancer. Processed soy foods were thought to be the new route to better health for a while, and then, with the exception of fermented soy foods, they were considered a health risk. Now the conversation has turned to getting large quantities of omega-3s, -6s, and -9s, along with antioxidants and vitamin D. Soon these will be old news and it will be something else.

AWARENESS

When we live our lives in a state of awareness, we can let go of many of the rules and concepts and simply live life as it happens. If we listen to our bodies and know from our own experiences which foods work best for us, then we don't need to be distracted by the swings of nutritional science.

Part of the journey into awareness is to be aware of change. All our senses function only through experiencing change. We can see only when there are different colors or light frequencies. If we walked into a room where everything was exactly the same color, we would not see anything. We become aware of sound when the pitch and frequencies changes. Without any changes in temperature, we would not be aware of hot and cold.

So we can be aware of how we feel as the day changes from morning to afternoon. How do we feel in the winter as compared to the summer? Do we react differently to rain and sun? What effect does a change in diet have on us? How do we feel after meditating on our breathing for few minutes? Can we detect a change in our moods and energies after exercising? Does chanting change our energies? If so, how does this compare to stretching?

It's through change that we experience life, and I would propose that by engaging in change, we can experience more in life. Embracing change is fundamentally the key ingredient for living a big life. Resisting change and getting stuck with wanting to hold onto beliefs that worked at one time in our lives potentially makes our lives smaller as we rule out so many options.

One of the effects of living in our own intuition is that we are freer to change with our world, as we don't have to struggle with beliefs that may hold us back. One of the themes of this book is living our lives with awareness of ourselves and everything around us, rather than getting stuck with other people's ideas—including mine!

RELATIVITY

Thoughts of relativity date back to Taoist and Greek philosophers, but for many people it was Albert Einstein who famously delivered his theory of relativity describing relativity in a scientific context. Einstein proposed that space, time, and gravity were not constant, but change according to their relationship to the observer.

The basic idea here is that there are no absolutes. We can only compare one thing to another. When driving our cars, we can compare our speed to the land around us and get one reading; if we compare our rate of movement to the other side of our planet or to the moon, we will get other readings. Similarly, we could not claim that a carrot is healthy, but only that it is healthier than candy. Even then, that might not always hold true; there may be circumstances when the candy is healthier than the carrot.

The Greek sophists used relativism to consider the role we have in our observation of our universe. Is what we see the same for someone else? Do we each have our unique experiences of the universe, and does this change according to our current conditions? Is what is true for us true for anyone else?

When we mix the idea of relativity with the claim that everything is in a constant state of change, we describe a universe that is fluid, soft, elastic, bendy, and stretchy. Even time and gravity change depending where we are in our cosmos. Somewhere in all of this is me, and if I am relative to all this change, and relativity to everything else defines me, then by definition I must be in some kind of state of flux. In theory, as soon as I think of anything as an absolute, such as that I need brown rice every day to be healthy, I am in a state of delusion.

PERSONAL CHANGE

It's one thing to roam our universe exploring change and relativity, but how does this affect our real lives, if at all? It is, after all, a choice. We can still choose to view life as a set of constants and absolutes, and our lives will not fall apart. The worst that will happen is that people who believe in change and relativity will think we are old-fashioned and deluded. We can create our own rules and beliefs, and we may live as long and be just as healthy as anyone else.

In my experience, accepting the idea of continuous change fills our lives with possibilities and opportunities. Just because something didn't work before doesn't mean it won't work tomorrow. We can change, evolve, and develop to be more successful. In many ways, this is a very positive, optimistic way of living. If Dragana and I get into a pattern of behavior in our relationship that does not make us happy, then we can both change it and evolve to a new way of relating that creates a more enjoyable relationship.

In a sense, every day is new and a fresh start. We have the ability to change at any time and create the lives we are looking for. We also have the ability to take on all kinds of healing; at any time we can change ourselves biologically, emotionally, and mentally.

Living in a world of change and relativity does take more effort. It's much easier to sit back with the familiar and live with constants than to embrace change and be open to being different. It's most likely that we will be spurred to change and evolve during difficult times, and the biggest challenge is to carry on the process when things are going well. In my experience of teaching macrobiotic philosophy and cooking, most people come because they feel a need to address health issues. Trying out a macrobiotic lifestyle could be just as helpful in life when someone is feeling well, but humans are less likely to make the effort when there is no obvious pressure.

Living a life of change and relativity also takes away all those assumptions that are based on consistency that can be so reassuring. The "always" and "never" disappear along with the "shoulds" and "shouldn'ts." When we accept constant change, we can live only in the moment, letting go of what happened yesterday or the day before, and not making assumptions or having expectations about what will happen tomorrow.

This is especially helpful is in relationships, where so much harm can come from making long-term assumptions about someone and expecting that he or she will carry on in the same way forever. Again, I would not claim that embracing change is a better way of living but a different way, and one that for some people can help throw off all those self-imposed restrictions, leading to huge new possibilities. For someone else it might create confusion, a loss of structure, and lack of boundaries.

CHANGES WITHIN MACROBIOTICS

It would be strange for a movement that advocates change not to change itself; consequently, macrobiotics has gone through and is still going through many changes. This can be confusing if you read a book on macrobiotics that was written thirty years ago and expect it to be the same as one written today. Before long, this book may seem out of date.

During the time I have been involved in macrobiotics, there have been quite few changes. Macrobiotics went through a stage when it was seen as a diet, and the common perception was that it was a highly restrictive way of eating, with a limited list of "allowed" foods.

Changes to the Macrobiotic Way of Eating

For many people, macrobiotics has become an awareness of their personal relationships with food and a greater general understanding of food, hopefully leading to being able to use their intuition more clearly in terms of food choices.

Other people still prefer to think of macrobiotics as being a diet, but even this has changed to include a bigger range of foods. Specifically, nightshade foods such as tomatoes, potatoes, and peppers that were once considered unhealthy but are now generally accepted as contributing to a healthy diet.

There was a time when fruit in general and especially raw fruit was thought to be too yin, cooling and weakening. Sweeteners like rice syrup were preferred because they come from grains, even though they are much higher on the glycemic index. Similarly, there was a general rule that everything should be cooked, with the exception of pickles and pressed salads. Raw salads did not figure into a typical macrobiotic diet. Many people eating macrobiotically now enjoy regular raw salads and fruits.

Through experience, long-term macrobiotics practitioners have found that they often need more processed grains than originally considered necessary. So breads, noodles, pasta, couscous, and polenta now form a greater part of many people's diets.

Macrobiotic teaching also fell into the thinking that polyunsaturated oils would be preferable to saturated fats in cooking; some macrobiotic teachers are revising this to recommend saturated fats and monounsaturated oils for cooking and polyunsaturated oils only for use when raw on salads and other foods. This would mean, for example, using olive oil for frying, butter for baking, and sunflower oil as part of a salad dressing.

In the past, the macrobiotic diet could be highly acid-forming. Most of the grains, beans, nuts, seeds, and fish are acid-forming; and only the vegetables and a few other foods are alkaline-forming, which made macrobiotic diet unbalanced. This would have been exacerbated if some practitioners drank coffee, drank alcohol, or smoked cigarettes regularly, as these are also acid-forming. From an acid and alkaline perspective, the macrobiotic approach to eating becomes healthier when we include a much bigger proportion of vegetables. Where it once was recommended to make vegetables twenty-five percent of our diet, in my opinion it would ideally be at least fifty percent.

Understandably, when George Ohsawa's students came to the West from Japan, they brought with them their traditional cuisine. Many of the seasonings were Japanese. These tended to be sodium-rich and could lead to a diet too high in salt as people tried to add flavor to their food. Later, the seasoning changed to include all the traditional European herbs along with garlic, oils, lemon juice, apple cider vinegar, and any other natural seasonings.

In terms of bringing up children, many of us have recognized that a restrictive diet is not really suitable for children. As children do not have a long-term history of eating foods that have proved to be harmful, and as they are physically active, the risks associated with a broader diet are very small. In most cases it's safer and healthier to ensure they have a varied and full range of foods, including lots of fresh, natural, whole foods, rather than to worry that they might have too much of something less healthy.

Changes to the Macrobiotic Philosophy

During the cancer-cure phase, the macrobiotic movement became more prescriptive, with set diets and specific recipes. This undermined our desire to educate and help people create their own awareness of food and health. There is now a general change toward education, guiding people, and working with people over a period of time to help create that awareness and understanding of food.

There is less of an emphasis among many current teachers of macrobiotics on food being the cause of and solution to all health issues, and a greater acceptance of the role of stress, emotions, and thinking. Rather than aiming to cure illness, there has been a shift to making the most of our lives and living the big life. This might result in someone feeling better and finding that a health problem has disappeared, but it is no longer the main reason for trying macrobiotics.

There was an emphasis on thinking that food influenced everything and was our salvation for everything. This idea was extended to emotions, relationships, and spirituality. This may have brought about an obsession with food in some people, and because of constant claims that certain foods would cause cancer, some people developed fears about those foods. In an attempt to prevent cancer, people might find themselves eating a very narrow diet and then, when eating something not on the list, feel guilty or like a failure. In retrospect, this approach was not healthy in a holistic sense; it may have set up a nocebo effect, where someone would be so fearful of eating the "wrong" food that they would actually increase the likelihood of it being harmful.

The emphasis on food also took people's attention away from other influences on health, and perhaps for this reason there was a lack of attention to exercise, cultivating healthy relationships, and exploring our emotions. There has been a steady shift toward getting a better balance in life and putting food in its more appropriate position as just one of many influences that can affect our well-being.

I have also noticed a steady move away from being caught up in the macrobiotic concepts and toward using our experience to gain insights into life, health, and healing. This may be a natural process as a group of enthusiasts mature; it might also be part of a collective desire to return to our more intuitive roots.

As an exercise, you can reflect on the changes you have made to your life so far and test yourself on whether there are things about yourself you would find hard to change in the future.

CHAPTER THIRTY-ONE
Living Energy

The idea that humans have a subtle electromagnetic energy running through them has been used in China for healing, and it forms part of their philosophy of life. Similar ideas can be found in traditional Indian and Japanese thinking. The practice is to see energy moving along paths called meridians, while the Indian perception is of seven energy centers called chakras. In Europe, Dr. Christoph Wilhelm Hufeland expounded on this idea of a living energy or life force running through all living beings.

The thought that we have a life force of our own and that the way this life force moves through us could be influential on our health and well-being has been an established part of macrobiotic thinking. In China, this life force is known as chi, and I have based this chapter partly on the traditional Chinese and Indian understandings, and partly on our modern interpretation.

CHI

Chi is a subtle electromagnetic energy that runs through everything we know. It carries information with it as it flows from one thing to another. The energy flowing through our bodies will predominantly carry our thoughts, beliefs, and emotions, but it also mixes with the energies around us.

You could imagine it as an energy field that runs through you and around you—a bit like a magnetic field. All the time, some of your energy is floating off, away from you, while you also draw in new energy from the ambient energy surrounding you.

This suggests that some of your thoughts and emotions literally float off into world around you. Somewhere out there will be the energy of your all your thoughts, emotions, and beliefs floating around our planet. This is sometimes referred to as mass consciousness. The idea is that everyone's ideas surround us and when you really relax you can tap into these thoughts and pick up interesting insights, and even solutions to your own problems.

The fresh chi you draw into your own energy field brings in something of the world around you. This could include the energy of the weather, people close to you, the atmosphere of your home, and the energy of the food you eat. As any of these energies enter your own energy field, they can alter your own chi makeup, resulting in you feeling different and having new thoughts.

In addition to the chi being radiated and absorbed by your body, you can change the energy within you. The clothes you wear, having a shower, doing some stretching, or having acupuncture all change your energy field and, again, make you feel and think differently. Most important, you can change your own energy with your thoughts and emotions. If you adopt a different perception of a situation, your energy will change and you will feel different. We can literally change our own energies regardless of all the other influences. For example, meditating on my breathing for a few seconds helps me quickly reach a content, peaceful state regardless of the weather, where I am, who I'm with, or what I've eaten.

CHAKRAS

The Indian view of our energetic bodies is that we have seven areas of intense activity of energy, known as chakras. Each chakra has a location and is associated with certain qualities. The following descriptions are useful to help understand the idea behind the chakras, but ultimately it is for you to experience the energy of your chakras for yourself.

Crown chakra, at the top of the head—exterior energy mixes with our own, linking us to the heavens. It is here that we are guided to evolve, grow, and develop.

Midbrain chakra, between the eyebrows—this energy is the center of the intellect and can be where the intuition resides.

Throat chakra, in the throat—focuses on expression and communication.

Heart chakra, between the nipples—it's through this chakra that we can access our souls and deepest feelings of love.

Stomach chakra, in the solar plexus—the center for willpower, aspiration, and determination.

Abdominal chakra, two finger widths below the navel—this represents the center of our power and vitality.

Reproductive chakra, behind the pubic bone—the energy here is associated with reproduction and primal instincts.

You can experiment by putting your hand over each of these chakras and practicing your gentle breathing meditation. Try leaving your hand on each chakra for a few minutes before moving on to the next chakra. Another option is to work with other person: Ask your friend to lie down and practice the breathing meditation while you put your hand on one of his or her chakras and go into the same breathing meditation. After a few minutes, move on to the next chakra.

As you do this, be aware of how you feel and use this awareness to get to know each of your chakras.

MERIDIANS AND ACUPRESSURE POINTS

Acupuncture is based on the idea that as your energy, or chi, flows through paths or meridians of energy; you can change it at specific points called acupressure points. The energy flowing through meridians is thought to spread out into smaller and smaller paths until it feeds every cell in our bodies. In this way it mirrors how our blood vessels bring blood to every cell.

Interestingly, there are fourteen meridians; some people assign two meridians to each chakra. You could think of chakras as wells of energy and meridians as rivers, streams, and brooks distributing energy.

There are just over 360 acupressure points located across the human body; these can be readily found in a book on shiatsu, acupressure, or Chinese medicine, as well as in my book *Chi Energy Workbook.*

You can locate many of the points by feeling along bones and looking for little sensitive indentations and ridges. Also, try between bones, like those on the top of your feet, and between muscles and bones. These are places that chi can get stuck, caught up, constrained, and stagnant. Similarly, if you press on the muscles you will often find sensitive points where there may be too much or too little energy.

Simply pressing and holding the point for a few seconds can be enough to help move energy again. You can also try tapping, massaging, or rubbing and see what feels most helpful to you.

FEEL ENERGY BETWEEN HANDS

Although you have chi flowing through your body, it's not always easy to access it and focus it strongly. The easiest way to concentrate and project your chi is through your hands, although you could use any part of your body.

Begin by finding a space that feels right to you. Perhaps somewhere with a natural atmosphere, free from electrical equipment, clutter, and synthetic materials. Choose a reasonably large space, such as one of your larger rooms or a secluded space outside. Wear loose cotton clothing and choose a time of day when you are least likely to be interrupted. In theory, you'll have the best results doing this at sunrise, barefoot, and outside so you can feed off the energy of the dew rising off the grass.

Stand up and rub your hands together vigorously until they feel warm all over. Rub the palms, backs, and sides of your hands. Next, rub the outside of your upper arms. Take one step forward, breath in, and stretch your hands upward while breathing out. Step back and let your arms drop to your sides. Step forward with the other foot and repeat the breathing and stretch. Do this at least three times, fully inflating your abdomen and chest, followed by a long out breath. Vigorously shake your hands, keeping your wrists and fingers relaxed and loose. Try to imagine you're shaking the blood right down to the tips of your fingers.

Hold the root of your thumb firmly between your other thumb and index finger, and massage all the way down to your thumbnail. Squeeze your thumb at each side of the nail base and breath in. Pull gently as you breathe out, and quickly move your thumb and index finger away from your thumb. As you do this, imagine you have a multicolored flame of energy around your thumb and that you are extending it. Repeat with each finger on the same hand and then repeat with the other hand.

Remain standing and put the palms of your hands together in front of your chest. Each time you breath in, imagine you are breathing a powerful color, feeling, or sound into your body. For example, breathe a strong red color, a warm feeling, or the roar of a lion deep into your abdomen. Choose whatever has the greatest effect on you. As you breathe out, imagine the powerful color, feeling, or sound moving up into your hands. Repeat this several times.

If the palms of your hands feel at all damp once you have completed this stage, dry them on a cotton cloth or your clothes. Give the palms a vigorous rub together for at least ten seconds. Now hold your hands about a foot or thirty centimeters apart, and start to move them closer and further apart. Be very sensitive to any feeling in the palms of your hands. Do the same with your hands further apart. Experiment, and play with gently moving your hands together and apart. Try moving very slowly, slightly quicker, small distances, and larger distances.

Bring your hands close together, and be aware of whether you feel the palms of your hands get slightly warmer. As you move your hands apart, you might feel this warmth continue, as though you are pulling this warm energy field further apart. Keep playing, letting your palms move into the warmer energy, and then pull the warm chi apart.

Then, close your eyes for greater sensitivity and focus your mind on your hands as you move them evenly together and apart. At this point, you may feel a slight magnetic sensation between your hands as they change from moving apart to moving toward each other.

If you don't feel anything at first, keep trying; the more you do this exercise, the greater your ability to sense chi becomes.

FEELING THE ENERGY OF THE BACK

Using the following process, you can test your ability to feel energy on the back, and then try some healing and retest to see if there's any difference.

The person who is going to receive the treatment first needs to lie on his or her stomach, with his or her back exposed to the base of the spine. To feel where your friend's energy is in excess or deficient, move the palm of your hand across your friend's back, about two inches or five centimeters away from the skin. As you do this, be aware of any areas that feel hot or cold. Be careful not to leave your hand in one place for too long, as you'll begin to connect with your friend's energy and he or she will start to change. Usually making one or two passes over your friend's back will be sufficient to make a quick intuitive reading. Remember the areas that felt warmer or cooler.

Next, drag the back of your thumbnails slowly down either side of your friend's spine. Hold your thumbnails at an angle of about forty-five degrees. You can usually press firmly. If you like, do a test on your forearm first so you can see how much pressure is comfortable, and then work with your friend. Watch your partner's back carefully, and you'll see two red lines start to appear. You'll notice that in some areas the line grows into a broad band, and in others it appears thin, or may not even turn red at all. The places where the line is broad and strongly colored have plenty of energy coming to the surface; those places where the line is thin show have energy that is more withdrawn.

Rest your hand on the area where the line is pale or thin, and relax into your breathing meditation for a few minutes. Wait until you feel a heat develop between your hand and your friend's back. Then, try making new lines next to the old while passing through the area where you've been resting your hand. Observe the lines and see if the areas you have connected with have produced a redder line.

If you are receiving this treatment, be aware of any changes you may notice in your emotions or physical feelings.

EXCHANGING ENERGY WITH ANOTHER PERSON

When people receive any kind of healing treatment, their bodies will cool down as they relax, with the result that they can feel cold. It's important to find a space that is warm and have blankets or towels around, so you can wrap up any parts of your friend's body that feel cold. The person receiving the treatment would ideally wear pure cotton garments to make it easier to feel a strong connection.

Begin by doing the exercises to generate chi in your hands. You'll need to spend a little time getting your energy centered and ready for the treatment.

Try initiating every in and out breath with your mind, while being aware of everything about the feeling of your breath. I suggest you try to complete your treatment in silence so you can fully concentrate on connecting with your friend.

The technique is to place the palms of your hands on your friend and meditate on your breathing. You can move your hands to positions where you intuitively feel the person needs to experience healing. Rest your hands for several minutes until you feel your palms heat up. You can keep one hand on the upper back, behind the heart chakra, or on the front on the upper chest, while you put your free hand in other positions.

Your contact can be light, just the weight of your hands, as the purpose is to connect energetically. To make this easy and relaxing for you, sit close to your friend and keep your shoulders comfortably close to the place to are working on. A comfortable posture is one where your upper arms hang straight down from your shoulders and your forearms lay straight out in front of you.

The treatment consists of moving your hands to various points on your friend's body. You'll find that some areas warm up quicker than others, and you may need to spend considerably more time on certain parts before the area heats up. The following is a short treatment that covers various areas.

To carry out the treatment, ask your friend to lie on his or her front. Make sure he or she is comfortable, as your friend will need to lie in one place for some time. Kneel or sit cross-legged next to your friend. The following description is as if you are sitting on his or her left, so for simplicity's sake I suggest choosing that position.

Begin by placing your left hand gently on your friend's upper back, and your right on the lower back. Meditate on your breathing and be sensitive to the feeling in your hands. You can raise them occasionally to see if you are developing a magnetic connection with your friend. Once you reach the point where you feel a heat in the palm of your hands, you can move on to the next location. I suggest you take your right hand away from the lower back very slowly, and hold your hand about two centimeters or an inch away from your friend's body for a while, encouraging chi to flow through the air. Interestingly, this part can create a more intense and active interchange of energy than when you are in direct contact. Sometimes your palms will heat up considerably at this point.

Next, place your right hand over one of your friend's kidneys. This will be just above the lowest rib, on the back and to the side of the spine. When you feel ready, gently move your hand to over the opposite kidney. Now you can move your hands so that your right rests on your friend's upper back and your left is on the back of your friend's neck. When your left hand has warmed, move it slowly up to the back of your friends head.

Ask your friend to turn over slowly. If he or she has fallen asleep, wake him or her gently. Now, place your left hand on his or her upper chest and your right between the hip bones and above the pubic bone. Remember to go back to your breathing meditation. When you feel ready, move your right hand up and place it over your friend's lower left ribs; then, once it feels appropriate, move your right hand and place it over your friend's right ribs.

Now you can move your hands again, placing your right hand on your friend's upper chest and your left hand on his or her forehead. You can complete your exchange by finally moving your left hand to the top of your friend's head.

After the treatment, let your friend relax and remain silent. This might be a good time to cover him or her with blanket so your friend can remain calm and let his or her energy settle.

THE LIFE FORCE IN FOODS

In my experience, the foods we eat contain a life force, living energy, or chi of their own. Every time we eat, some of the energy of the food enters our bodies and mixes with our own energies. For me, the influence is greater when eating whole living foods. It's particularly noticeable with raw vegetables and fruits, but it can also be felt with cooked whole foods such as whole grains, dried beans, and cooked vegetables.

In theory, all foods will contain some form of energy, but in processed foods the energy is often too confused for us to be able to feel and distinguish it. To feel the energy of foods, be aware of how you feel and your emotions immediately after eating. The energy of a food will have an almost immediate effect on your energy, whereas the nutritional content can take an hour or more to bring about any kind of biological change.

To feel the energy of a food, begin by using your gentle breathing meditation to reach a calm, empty state of stillness and awareness. Then consume the food and repeat your meditation. Just be aware of the changes you experience in your energy and make a note. For example, I could meditate for a minute or two, eat an apple, and then do the same meditation. I might then be aware of greater mental clarity, increased energy levels, and a slight cool feeling in my abdomen. After a while I could do the same exercise with a banana and be aware of the differences between the two fruits.

By eating with this kind of awareness, over time we will attune ourselves to the way we react to the different kinds of energy in foods. Some will feel cooling and others warming, some will seem to stimulate us mentally while others strengthen our abdomens, and we might feel that some foods nurture our hearts and others our stomachs. Sometimes a food will feel as though it speeds up the movements of our energy, and then another food slows them down. You may feel that some foods spread your energy to the surface of your skin while others help you build up your inner strength. It may be that some foods feel like they move your energy toward your feet, and some help move your energy toward your head.

I would encourage you to experience this for yourself and be aware of your relationship to your food, rather than using someone else's lists of how the living energy of different foods might influence your energy. Remember that the influence of any food is subtle, and you can redirect and control your own energy regardless of what you eat; however the energy of some foods will help you feel that ability to control your own energy.

SUGGESTIONS FOR BEING MORE AWARE OF ENERGY

The following are suggestions for helping you feel more sensitive to your own energy and the influences on your energy. I suggest you try these ideas for a month or two.

1. Eat whole, living foods that are high in living chi energy.
2. Wear clothes that are made of cotton or other natural materials.
3. Try to work, relax, or sleep at least a meter or yard from any electrical equipment.
4. Make sure your bedding is made from pure cotton and that your home has as many natural materials as possible.
5. Exercise and stretch in a place that has a natural feel to it several times a week.
6. Meditate on your breathing daily.
7. Go out into nature frequently.

CHAPTER THIRTY-TWO
Acid and Alkaline

Sagen Ishizuka and George Ohsawa made the balance of acid and alkaline a key issue in macrobiotics, and Herman Aihara went on to write his acclaimed book *Acid and Alkaline* to examine it in detail.

Sagen Ishizuka claimed that people generally suffer poor health from overacidity rather than from being too alkaline. When eating more alkaline-forming foods, the body stores minerals; when your body is too acidic, these minerals are used up as your body tries to maintain an optimum pH balance in the blood. This is thought to aggravate arthritic conditions and could lead to a weakening of the bones as phosphorus is taken from them. A generally acidic condition is also thought to increase the risk of cancer and headaches, and to reduce our resistance to infectious illnesses.

So far it's not known how much the pH of our intercellular fluid changes in response to outside influences. We know our saliva and urine change their pH in response to outside influences, but the rest is speculation. From my own experience, maintaining a condition where my saliva is consistently alkaline has helped me feel healthier in terms of my energy, immune system, and joints.

When we feel stressed we tend to secrete more acid into our digestive system with the result that our saliva, urine, and, possibly, other body fluids become more acidic. This may be one reason why humans become more prone to illness when suffering from long term stress. There are many claims that illnesses like cancer, psoriasis, shingles, headaches, indigestion, ulcers, rheumatoid arthritis and heart disease are more likely to occur during times of prolonged stress. It is also though we are more susceptible to infectious illness whilst feeling stressed. In my own work many clients connect the start of an illness with a period of great stress. So we might hypothesize that stress contributes to more acidic condition and that over acidity can result in poor health in some people.

In addition to stress, certain foods can lead to us becoming more acidic. These are known as acid-forming foods. Interestingly, some foods that are themselves acidic, such as lemons, actually result in a more alkaline condition in our saliva and urine. There are different ways of measuring foods in terms of their pH. Some tables are based on burning foods and analyzing their ashes, others measure a person's urine or saliva at the peak of the wave of change the foods bring about.

The pH value derived from burning food tells us more about the possible effect of the food in our digestive systems, and the test that measures the foods effect on our saliva and urine provides more clues as to the effect it may have on some of our other bodily fluids. For example, drinking lemon juice will feel acidic in our mouths and stomachs, and often make an overly acidic condition such as an ulcer worse, whereas it could be helpful for a headache caused by overacidity.

In addition, the health of your digestive system can have an influence on whether foods become acid- or alkaline-forming. For example, tomatoes are considered slightly alkaline-forming but they become acid-forming when stomach acid is low or thyroid activity is subnormal. In addition, the more mature and ripe the tomato, the more alkaline-forming it becomes. It is therefore difficult to produce a reliable table. I use a broad spectrum of tables based on foods' possible influence on the body as a rough guide to acid- and alkaline-forming foods, and then use pH sticks to measure my own saliva.

In what is often thought of as a typical macrobiotic diet based on whole, living foods, most grains and beans will be acid-forming, while vegetables and many fruits are alkaline-forming. This is why it is important to generally have as much vegetables as you have grains in a typical day. If you add in fish, salty dairy foods, and meat, your diet becomes more acid-forming, increasing the need for vegetables and fruits. Cigarettes, coffee, and alcohol make your diet even more acid-forming. A typical junk food diet is highly acid-forming.

The starting point to creating a balanced diet in terms of acid and alkaline is to have roughly equal amounts of grains and vegetables, and then try to match additional acid-forming foods with an increase in alkaline-forming foods. For example if you eat more fish, reduce your intake of grains slightly and increase your intake of vegetables or fruits. Try having alkaline-forming lemon or chopped almonds with your fish. If you enjoy alcohol sometimes, try to also eat more alkaline-forming foods. Have an alkaline-forming fresh vegetable juice with the occasional coffee.

To increase the alkaline-forming foods within your diet, try a miso soup with a variety of vegetables and wakame, dulse, or nori daily. Adding celery, watercress, and parsley to your soup will make it much more alkalizing. Use a little more millet and reduce other grains, make a drink by squeezing lemon into a glass and poring hot water over it, have fresh melon for desert, cook parsley as a vegetable dish, try tofu instead of beans more often, drink kukicha or herbal teas, and have freshly squeezed vegetable or fruit juices.

The following is a list of what are generally considered to be acid- and alkaline-forming foods. I would highly recommend testing your own saliva regularly to get your own experience of what it takes to keep yourself in a more alkaline condition. Remember to combine this with adequate relaxation, meditation, and laughter. In the end, it's how you feel that matters, and the ultimate test will be to listen to your body and see for yourself if you can sense any difference when according to your saliva test you are in a more alkaline state.

Most Alkaline-Forming

Agar agar, cayenne, celery, dates (dried), figs (dried), herb teas (most types), kudzu root, lemons, limes, mango, melons, papaya, parsley, all seaweeds, grapes, watercress.

Moderately Alkaline-Forming

Alfalfa sprouts, almonds, apple cider vinegar, apples, apricots, asparagus, avocados, bananas (ripe), bancha/kukicha tea, beans (fresh, green), beets, bell peppers, broccoli, cabbage, carob, cauliflower, chard, currants, daikon, dates (fresh), figs (fresh), fruit juices (with pulp and without sugar), garlic, ginger (fresh), grapefruit, green tea, herbs, kale, kiwis, lettuce, nectarines, passionfruit, peaches, pears, peas (fresh), pickled vegetables (homemade/natural), pineapple, potatoes (with skins), pumpkin, radishes, raisins, raspberries, shiitake mushrooms, spring greens, strawberries, squash, sweet corn (fresh), sweet potatoes, turnips, *umeboshi,* vegetable juices.

Slightly Alkaline-Forming

Almonds, brown rice syrup, brown rice vinegar, brussels sprouts, buckwheat, cherries, chestnuts (dry, roasted), coconut (fresh), cucumbers, eggplant, Essene bread, goat's milk (unhomogenized), honey (raw), Jerusalem artichokes, leeks, miso, mushrooms, okra, olives, olive oil, onions, oranges, sea salt, sesame seeds (whole), shoyu, soybeans (dry), soy cheese, soy milk, spices, sprouted grains (most types), tamari, tangerines, tempeh, tofu, tomatoes, wild rice.

Close to Neutral

Butter (unsalted), cream (fresh, raw), cow's milk (unhomogenized), millet, oils (except olive), yogurt (plain), whey (raw).

Slightly Acid-Forming

Barley, barley malt, butter (salted), eggs, kidney beans, pumpkin seeds, spelt, spinach, sprouted wheat breads.

Moderately Acid-Forming

Beans (dried; except soybeans), blueberries, bran, bread (made from sprouted organic wheat), cheese, coconut (dried), cow's milk (homogenized), eggs (hard-cooked), fish, fructose, goat's milk (homogenized), grains (unrefined), honey (pasteurized), ketchup, maple syrup (unprocessed), molasses (unsulphured and organic), mustard, nuts (most, except almonds), oats, pasta (whole grain), pastry (made with whole grains and honey), plums, popcorn (with salt and/or butter), potatoes (peeled), prunes, rice (basmati and brown), rice milk, rye, seeds, tea, venison.

Most Acid-Forming

Alcohol (most forms), artificial sweeteners, beef, beer, bread (made from whole or refined wheat), carbonated soft drinks, cereals (refined), chocolate, cigarettes and other tobacco products, coffee, cranberries, cream of wheat (unrefined), custard (made with white sugar), drugs, fish, flour (refined wheat), fruit juices with sugar, ice cream, jams, jellies, lamb, maple syrup (processed), molasses (sulphured), pasta (white), pastries (made with white flour and/or sugar), peanuts, pickles (commercial), pork, poultry, rice (white), salt (refined and iodized), seafood, sugar, walnuts, white vinegar (processed), wine, yogurt (sweetened).

CHAPTER THIRTY-THREE
Glycemic Index

The time it takes for our food to influence our blood sugar levels has a great influence on our health. This is important because frequent, rapid changes in blood sugar increase the risk of developing type two diabetes, and can eventually contribute to heart disease and strokes in some people. Some scientists have even associated blood sugar fluctuations with an increased risk of cancer.

In addition, people often find that a rapid increase in blood sugar is followed by a blood sugar low, as the initial rise causes the pancreas to release insulin; the body then reduces blood sugar levels by storing the excess sugars. A blood sugar low can result in cravings for more foods with a high sugar content, leading to a situation where a person's blood sugar rises and falls dramatically throughout the day. It is common for people falling into this pattern to put on excess weight. Many people have found it easier to lose weight by eating foods that encourage their blood sugar to rise slowly, which reduces the risk of craving sweets and subsequently converting sugar to fat.

Knowing which foods will maintain stable blood sugar levels is essential for anyone trying to control diabetes through diet. For this reason it is helpful to rank foods according to the rate at which they change blood sugar levels. Dr. David Jenkins at St. Michael's Hospital in Toronto first studied and created the glycemic index (GI), which proved to shed surprising new light on which foods actually have the greatest effect on our blood sugar levels.

The GI is a system of measuring how quickly eating different carbohydrate-rich foods increases blood sugar levels. The higher the number, the quicker the blood sugar response; so a low-GI food will cause a slow rise, while a high-GI food will trigger a dramatic blood sugar spike, often followed by a blood sugar low. A GI of seventy or more is high, a GI of between fifty-six and sixty-nine is medium, and a GI of fifty-five or less is considered low.

The glycemic load (GL) is another way to assess the impact of carbohydrate consumption that takes the glycemic index into account, but gives a fuller picture. A GI value tells you only how rapidly the carbohydrate component of a particular food turns into sugar. It doesn't tell you how much of the carbohydrate is in a serving of a particular food. You need to know both things to understand a food's effect on blood sugar. For example, the carbohydrate in watermelon has a high GI, but because there's not a lot of it, watermelon's glycemic load is relatively low. A GL of twenty or more is high, a GL between eleven and nineteen is medium, and a GL of ten or less is low.

The idea of maintaining stable blood sugar levels has long been an important aim of macrobiotic practitioners; in this sense, macrobiotics could be claim to be the original GI diet. Foods with a GI of fifty-five or less are considered ideal, and, looking through the table below, you will see most whole, living macrobiotic foods have a GI of fifty-five or less. The exceptions to this are millet, apricots, raisins, watermelon, broad beans, pumpkin, beets, potatoes, sweet potatoes, and rutabagas. You also need to consider the amount of carbohydrate a food will convert into blood sugar, the glycemic load or GL. If the GL is ten or less, it is considered low, so foods like apricots, watermelon, broad beans, pumpkin, beets, and rutabagas may increase your blood sugar quickly, but do not raise it particularly far, as there are not sufficient carbohydrates in a typical serving.

From a macrobiotic perspective there's another issue, and that is the effect of taking in the energies of these high GI or GL foods and the influence of unstable blood sugar levels on our emotions. As our blood sugar reaches a high, it is common to feel hyperactive, unfocused and slightly out of control, while during a blood sugar low it becomes easier to feel depressed, pessimistic, and drained. Rapidly changing blood sugar levels seems to particularly affect children, precipitating tantrums, later followed by feeling withdrawn.

Looking through the information and tables below, interesting patterns emerge.

1. Whole grains have a lower GI than processed grains. For example, white rice has a GI of sixty-four, while brown rice registers at fifty-five.
2. You can reduce the GI of brown rice by mixing it with another low-GI grain such as whole barley.

3. Puffed grains like rice cakes or puffed rice cereals have a much higher GI than the original whole grain.

4. The longer a food is cooked, the higher the GI. For example, the natural sugars in pasta cooked al dente are absorbed more slowly than when pasta is overcooked. Spaghetti boiled in salted water for eleven minutes has a GI of fifty-nine, while boiling for sixteen minutes gives it a GI of sixty-five.

5. Most vegetables, beans, nuts and seeds have a GI that is too low to be considered significant.

6. Baking or frying foods raises their GI. Potatoes have a GI of eighty-five when baked, seventy-five when fried, and fifty when boiled.

7. Fish, eggs, and meat have GIs that are too low to be considered relevant.

The glycemic index is complicated and cannot be generalized to all people. Different people will have different reactions to food. Your body's response to food will vary according to several factors, including your age, activity level, insulin levels, and metabolism; the time of day you're eating; the amount of fiber and fat in the food; whether the food has been processed; what you ate along with the food; the ratio of carbohydrates to fat and protein; and how the food was cooked.

For example, a child running around outdoors will burn of blood sugar quickly, whereas an adult sitting in a warm office will not. Food high in GI or GL will not necessarily affect an active child. So while these tables are an interesting guide to how different foods can affect us, and while they can be useful for anyone wishing to lose weight or moderate their moods, they are not recommended as the sole basis for choosing foods.

My own experience has been that eating whole foods greatly improves my endurance, consistency of mood, and emotional stability. With whole, unprocessed foods, I find it easier to maintain my ideal weight and go through the day without cravings for snacks. For these reasons I would prefer to have fruit, nuts, or seeds than a healthy cookie or energy bar. By simply focusing on predominantly whole, unprocessed food, my diet naturally becomes low in terms of its GI and GL.

As always, it's for you to try out and see for yourself how you feel after a few weeks of choosing foods a certain way.

This chart uses glucose as its reference (glucose = 100).

	GI Glucose=100	Serving grams	GL Per serving
Juices			
Apple juice, unsweetened	41	250	12
Carrot juice, freshly made	43	250	10
Orange juice	50	250	13
Grains			
Baguette (white, plain)	95	30	15
Rye kernel bread	50	30	6
Bread (white, wheat)	70	30	10
Whole grain bread	71	30	9
Pita bread (white)	57	30	10
Swiss muesli	56	30	9
Porridge (whole oats)	51	250	11
Porridge (oat flakes)	55	250	15
Barley (pot or pearled whole)	25	150	11
Buckwheat	54	150	16
Cornmeal/polenta	69	150	9
Millet	71	150	25
Rice (white)	64	150	23
Rice (basmati)	58	150	22
Rice (brown)	55	150	18
Rye (whole, dry)	34	50	13
Linguine (durum wheat)	46	180	21
Rice noodles	61	180	23
Spaghetti (white)	57	180	27
Spaghetti (whole grain)	37	180	16
Rice cakes	78	25	17

	GI Glucose=100	Serving grams	GL Per serving
Dairy			
Yogurt	36	200	3
Fruit			
Apples	38	120	6
Apricots	57	120	5
Bananas	52	120	12
Grapes	49	120	9
Kiwis	53	120	6
Oranges	42	120	5
Peaches	42	120	5
Pears	38	120	4
Plums	39	120	5
Raisins	64	60	28
Strawberries	40	120	1
Watermelon	72	120	4
Beans (dried)			
Blackeyed peas	42	150	13
Lima beans	31	150	6
Chickpeas	28	150	8
Green beans	38	150	12
Kidney beans	28	150	7
Lentils (brown, red, and green)	30	150	5
Mung beans	42	150	7
Pinto beans	39	150	10
Soybeans	18	150	1
Snacks			
Corn chips	63	50	17
Cashews	22	50	3

	GI Glucose=100	Serving grams	GL Per serving
Snacks			
Peanuts	14	50	1
Hummus	6	30	0
Sweeteners			
Honey (pure)	58	25	12
Vegetables			
Fava beans	79	80	9
Peas	48	80	3
Pumpkin	75	80	3
Sweet corn	54	80	9
Beets	64	80	5
Carrots	47	80	3
Potatoes (baked)	85	150	26
Potatoes (boiled)	50	150	14
Potatoes (fried)	75	150	22
Sweet potatoes	61	150	17
Rutabagas	72	150	7

Most vegetables have too low a GI to consider. For example, artichokes, avocados, asparagus, bok choy, broccoli, brussels sprouts, cabbage, carrots, cauliflower, celery, cucumbers, eggplant, green beans, green peas, leeks, lettuce, mushrooms, onions, olives, peppers, spinach, squash, tomatoes, yams, and zucchini all have GIs of less than 55.

CHAPTER THIRTY-FOUR
Yin and Yang

Yin and yang describe how we can be connected to our universe. For example, the experience of climbing a mountain in the sun could be described as yang compared to the feelings we experience while lying in the shade. We can use yin and yang to describe our relationships with anything, including food, exercise, and the weather. Where it becomes interesting is that we can also describe our current state in terms of yin and yang. So I could say, "I feel really yin today." If I was not happy in that state, I could simply connect more deeply with those things I have identified with as helping me feel more yang, and change my current condition to being less yin.

Ultimately, yin and yang are wonderful ways to generate greater self-awareness and make interesting connections between our own conditions and all our possible interactions with the world we live in. Yin and yang allow us to connect ourselves to everything around us so that we can quickly decide what we need to do to bring ourselves back to a more balanced state when feeling any discomfort.

A very primitive use of the Chinese characters for yin and yang is thought to date back to the fourteenth century BC. It is thought that initially the character for yin described the night and yang the day. The *I Ching* explains a method of divination for receiving advice and insights from the divine, or our own subconsciouses, depending on your view, and in this book the broken lines that make up the hexagrams are considered yin and the solid lines yang. The *I Ching* is thought to have originated around 2800 BC, although it was also added to and developed later. A much more evolved interpretation of yin and yang appears throughout the *Yellow Emperor's Classic of Internal Medicine,* which was written anywhere between 2600 BC and 200 BC.

Yin and yang can be interpreted in different ways. For much of its history yin would describe the way we feel during the night and in winter compared to the yang feelings we might experience in the summer and during the day. In

Chinese medicine, the word "cooling" is associated with yin and "warming" with yang. So a food that feels warming would be more yang than a food that feels cooling.

George Ohsawa used expanding and contracting spirals to define his version of yin and yang, going back to an early interpretation as described by Fu Hsi. So a food that felt expanding, such as alcohol, would be classified as yin and a food the felt contracting, such as a dry, salty cracker, would be classified as yang. It is helpful to be aware that some things that are classified as yin in the current Chinese system are yang in George Ohsawa's version.

The basic idea of using two words to describe the effect of outside influences on us, and to cultivate the awareness of how we can help change our health through a change of those influences, works regardless of what definition we use. In one sense it's simply like learning a language. As my colleague Michael Rossoff points out, if we can speak the recent Chinese version of yin and yang, we communicate with a wide group of people also using yin and yang. The Chinese interpretation of yin and yang is used in feng shui, Chinese astrology, the *I Ching,* traditional Chinese medicine, acupuncture, Chinese herbal medicine, shiatsu, tai chi, qi gong, and Chinese philosophy. In this book I will use definitions familiar to the current Chinese system, which will have the added advantage of combining easily with the five elements explored in the next chapter.

One traditional Chinese interpretation is that yang is experienced on the sunny side of the mountain and yin on the shady side. Other ways we can experience natural environmental yin and yang is to see how we feel during a hot, dry, day in the summer, when there is a greater presence of yang energy compared to a cold, damp, frosty night in the winter. We could also compare the way we feel during the full moon to the new moon. During the full moon some of us become slightly more yang, and this corresponds with a three to five percent increase in car accidents, crime, and admissions to emergency rooms.

Using this definition of yin and yang, I would feel more energetic, expressive, outgoing, social, alert, warm, active, and motivated when I sense I am more yang. When I describe myself as more yin, I feel more withdrawn, introspective, meditative, cool, relaxed, calm, peaceful, objective, clear-minded, and insightful. I would suggest you make your own list of what feels like yin or yang to you, drawing on your experience of night and day, winter and summer, and shade and sun.

We are always more yin or yang and most of the time, and this is healthy; however, sometimes we may find we experience problems from being too yin or yang. Once we have identified whether we are too yang or yin, we can simply expose ourselves to more of the opposite energy and reduce the influences we have too much of. For example, if I felt too hot and active and this was contributing to a headache, as though the sun and heat was too strong for me, I could eat all the foods I know cool me down. For me, this would be raw cucumber, grated daikon, fresh fruits, lemon water, apple cider vinegar, plain yogurt, and salads. As a result, I would feel more yin; in the past, this has resulted in my headache receding.

To work out which foods tend to help you feel more yin or yang, be aware of how you feel after eating and see if the feeling you get from eating certain foods could be described in terms of feeling more wintry or summery. Do some foods help conjure up the feeling of being in the sun while others feel like sitting in the shade? It is important not to think of the foods you actually eat in the winter or summer, as these typically have the opposite influence.

You might find that the foods that most help you cool down and feel more like the night and winter are the foods you typically eat more during the summer. Similarly, the warming foods that encourage feeling summery may be the foods you eat more of during the winter. Without realizing it, we naturally try to find some kind of balance by eating more yin foods in summer and yang foods in winter.

Next time you feel unwell, try to identify how you feel and whether you feel more like the summer or winter to decide whether you are too yin or yang. Once you know your condition, try eating all the foods you would associate with the opposite. So if I felt tired and realized I felt kind of wintry inside, I could eat some of my warming foods that help me feel more like summer again.

It's helpful to remember that yin and yang are relative terms, not absolutes. For example, playing football might be a more yang experience than walking for me, but I also find walking a more yang experience than stretching. We are thinking in different shades of gray rather than in black and white.

Yin and yang can be applied to literally anything, and that is one of their greatest benefits. In macrobiotic practice, different foods and cooking styles are used to create meals that help our energy feel more yin or yang. Generally, raw foods or lightly cooked, watery vegetables help me feel more yin, and well-cooked dishes like porridge, casseroles, thick soups, stews, and fried foods help me feel more yang. The most warming foods like baked stews and pies can feel like they have the most yang influence.

My observation is that humans love to categorize, create rules, and make lists. It is therefore tempting to make lists of everything, sorting from yin to yang. I have done this myself many times in the past. The advantage is that we quickly get to see how it all can work in real life, but the disadvantage is that we could end up operating out of someone else's yin and yang list. Sometimes we can become highly conceptual, making a subject like yin and yang intellectual, agonizing over ancient Chinese texts and different interpretations. This takes us away from feeling yin and yang, into our heads and toward wanting to create man-made rules for ourselves. The risk is that we make our lives smaller as a result, and even alter or restrict our eating in a way that is not healthy and suppresses our natural intuition.

I have written out my own experience of yin and yang below so you can observe how I use it; you are welcome to use this as a guide to get started, but I would encourage you not to see these lists as somehow fixed or rigid—they are just my experience. Yours might be different, and I would encourage you to create your own feel for yin and yang, and to create your own lists if you feel like it.

TOO YIN

These are symptoms I would associate with feeling too yin: feeling cold; getting frequent infectious illnesses; having cold, clammy skin; having diarrhea; being lethargic; feeling depressed; and having a victim mentality.

TOO YANG

These are symptoms I would associate with feeling too yang: feeling hot; feeling irritable; having dry, itchy skin; having dry mouth; being stressed; being angry; and obsessing about details.

CHANGE TOWARD THE OPPOSITE

If I identify that I am predominantly yin or yang at a certain moment and I do not like the feeling, I try taking in more of the opposite energy by doing activities listed below. For example, if I thought I was too yin then I would try doing more from the "to become more yang" list.

To become more yin: meditate; eat more fresh fruit and salads; drink more water and juices; wear pastel colors; wear loose, flowing clothes; stretch; get out into nature; listen to relaxing music; light candles at night.

To become more yang: exercise; play competitive sports; wear bright colors; socialize; eat more cooked foods, root vegetables, grains, and fish; make to-do lists and structure the day.

REDUCE THE POSSIBLE CAUSES

At the same time, I can reduce the influences that might be causing me to feel too yin or yang using the lists below. Here, if I feel too yin I would apply the suggestions under "to become less yin."

To become less yin, reduce: consumption of ice cream, cold foods, raw fruit, and salads; regular use of alcohol; spending time sitting around; spending time watching television; spending time alone; exposure to a damp, cold climate; feeling powerless to change circumstances; blaming other people; waiting for someone else sort everything out.

To become less yang, reduce: consumption of baked foods, dry snacks, strong spices, and coffee; binge drinking of alcohol; exercise without stretching; setting standards that are too high; being obsessive; rushing; taking on too much; engaging in competitive activities.

Some foods can initially have a yang influence and then, later, a yin effect. For example, in the past, when I would drink alcohol at a party, I would initially feel warm, energized, and social—I would say more yang. However, drinking alcohol regularly also used to result in me feeling lethargic, tired, and even depressed—all attributes I would describe as coming from feeling too yin.

Similarly, sugar can give me a rush of energy, warmth, and a general yang feeling, only to make me feel cold and tired when my blood sugar drops. Strong spices can create a very recognizable yang feeling of burning and heat, and yet, eaten on a regular basis, they bring our heat to the surface so we can lose it through sweating, leaving us more cold and yin inside.

Sometimes a food or activity might have a very subtle effect on me in terms of yin and yang, but then, over a period of time, it this slowly accumulates to create stronger imbalances. For example, asking our children to do their homework does not really affect me, but if I start to let it become an everyday issue and even become obsessed with it, then I notice I start to feel more yang about their homework.

CHAPTER THIRTY-FIVE

The Five Elements

HISTORY

It's most likely that the five-elements theory started with the ancient Chinese calendar, in which five types of energy were assigned to different days, months, and years. The energies were given the names of five elements: wood, fire, earth, metal, and water. Each had a yin and a yang version, creating a ten-day week. The week would start with a yang wood day, followed by a yin wood day, yang fire day, yin fire day, yang earth day, yin earth day, yang metal day, yin metal day, yang water day, and, finally, a yin water day.

These five elements were associated with the equinoxes and solstices to help farmers plan ahead and organize their agricultural cycles. As you can imagine, having a calendar was of incredible benefit to an emerging agricultural civilization. The calendar was arranged using the elements: wood for the spring equinox, fire for the summer solstice, metal for the autumn equinox, and water for the winter solstice. The fifth element, earth, was at the centre of the calendar.

The relationships of humans to the cycles of the day, seasons, and moon were of interest to traditional Chinese physicians, and the five-element theory became a fundamental part of traditional healing. Early writing on the five elements can be found in the *Yellow Emperor's Classic of Internal Medicine.* Here, in a medical context, the five elements are arranged into a circle; unlike in the calendar, earth is part of the circle, placed between fire and metal.

The principles of the five elements became widespread and are fundamental to practices such as acupuncture, feng shui, shiatsu, qi gong, astrology, and healing through foods.

EXPERIENCE THE ENERGY OF EACH OF THE FIVE ELEMENTS

It's helpful to remember that the elements are just names used to describe five different types of energy. They are not the energy itself. The easiest way to experience the energy is to go out into nature at the appropriate time of year and day. There you can be aware of your experience of nature and how it influences you in terms of your emotions, thoughts, and feelings.

Wood

Walk barefoot in the grass early on a March morning to feel the dew rise and watch the sunrise. In the past I have felt the energy rise around me. Note your feelings at the beginning of the day. For example, I might feel enthused and ready to move forward into the new day.

Fire

Relax in the midday sun in June and be aware of flowers in bloom, colors, radiant heat, brightness, and activity. I often become aware of my own energy moving to the surface, and my experience of this is to feel more expressive, outgoing, and social.

Earth

Walk with the soil underfoot in the afternoon during July or August and be aware of the sun moving down in the sky. Note the fruits ripening on the vine, nature moving from growth to sweetness. I have felt cozy, comfortable, secure, or even like having a nap in this atmosphere.

Metal

Watch the sun set over the water in September and note the sun contracting as she dips below the horizon. Be aware of the end-of-the-day feelings and see if they bring sensations of contentment or satisfaction. Is there a sense of joy or pleasure?

Water

Go out into nature at night in December. Pick a clear night so you can see the stars and the universe above you. I might be deeply aware of myself and yet at the same time conscious of the vastness of the cosmos. I usually experience a stillness, peace, and tranquility in which I can find a new perspective on a problem.

THE CYCLE

In terms of yin and yang, we go from the night, December, and water energy being yin through to the rising yang energy of the sunrise, spring and wood energy, and then on to the yang of the midday, summer, and fire energy. Then we begin the yin phase of the cycle. During the yang phase, the sun is rising, the weather is getting hotter, plants are growing, and nature becomes more active. After the summer there is a phase of ripening. Vegetables and fruits get sweeter rather than growing, and the sun descends through the sky. The yin phase starts with earth energy and continues through the metal energy of the sunset and autumn, before changing again into the water, winter, and night phase.

You can make interesting observations on how humans respond to these cycles. For example, I often feel active and motivated in the morning. I also have similar feelings in the spring, when I am often inspired to take on new projects. The spring is a popular time to go on a diet or take up a new heath regime. We could say these begin to describe the character of wood energy.

Fire energy is associated with summer and the middle of the day; I often associate this with feeling social. The summer is a common time for festivals, social gatherings, and parties. This corresponds to lunchtime, when I might go out to meet people and make it a social part of my day. These observations suggest to me that fire energy helps me feel more expressive, outgoing, and social.

After lunch, I might feel sleepy and have a rest. This corresponds with July and August, when many people in the Northern Hemisphere choose to take a holiday. From our observations, we could claim that earth energy has a component that relates to rest, consolidation, and inactivity.

In many societies, the educational program starts close to the autumn equinox in September. This metal energy time also corresponds to the sun setting, when we might traditionally be finishing work. From my experience, I associate metal energy with education and developing myself, taking my energy inward, along with completing the day and completing projects.

During the night, I sleep and regenerate to get ready for the next day. During winter, nature does much the same thing. For me, winter is a time when I like to stay inside more and prepare for the year ahead. This can be an interesting time for self-reflection and exploring new possibilities for the year ahead.

If we stay with the five elements in terms of agriculture, then the elements follow each other in the order of wood/spring, fire/early summer, earth/late summer, metal/autumn, water/winter—and then wood again as the cycle repeats. This is considered a harmonious reflection of nature. However, if one of the five elements is weak, then the following element or phase of the agricultural growing cycle will be disturbed.

HEALTH

In people, a disruption of our five-element energies increases the risk of emotional disturbances and, eventually, a disturbed pattern of flow in our life energies. In theory, this might lead to a predisposition to certain ailments. In Chinese medicine, each element is associated with a pair of organs and different kinds of emotions. The emotions described in classical texts are what we would consider to be negative emotions; below I have added other typical characteristics.

Each element is also associated with a direction according to the movement of the sun at the time of day that an element is associated with. For example, wood is associated with the sunrise in the east, and the flow of energy is upward. In addition, each of the five elements is considered to have a taste that most closely represents its energy flow. Here are the traditional organs, emotions, potential health benefits, and tastes associated with each element. You can use these as a launching pad for developing your own experience and understanding of the five elements. In my experience, they are interesting for reflection and playing with our relationships with our environment.

Element	Time of Day	Season	Direction	Organs	Emotions	Health benefits	Taste
Wood	sunrise	spring	upward	liver and gallbladder	anger, impatience, activity; positive attitude, enthusiasm	increased energy	sour
Fire	midday	summer	outward	heart and small intestine	hysteria, excitement, expressive, outgoing social feelings	improved circulation and energy brought to the surface	bitter
Earth	afternoon	late summer	downward	spleen, pancreas, and stomach	jealousy; quality of life, practicality, stability, homeliness	strengthened digestive system	sweet
Metal	evening	autumn	inward	lungs and colon	depression, playfulness, contentment, containment	inner strength	umami (this is a kind of savory, fermented taste)
Water	night	winter	flowing in any direction	kidneys and bladder	fear, objectivity, creativity, originality, flexibility	physical and sexual vitality	salty

MACROBIOTICS AND THE FIVE ELEMENTS

In the macrobiotic application of the five elements, we can look to see if a deficiency or excess of one of the elements could be contributing to a physical or emotional issue, and then experiment to see if we can resolve this by making adjustments to our diets.

To do this, we need to think of foods in terms of which of the five-element energies they might increase inside our bodies. This is open to interpretation, but here are my suggestions, with a few examples. You can create your own list by feeling the effect of foods in terms of the seasons, and seeing which season and element best represents the way each food feels inside you.

Wood: leafy green vegetables either raw, steamed, or boiled for a minute or less; sauerkraut; vinegar; and lemons.

Fire: fried onions, garlic, ginger, spring onions, or scallions; mild spices; coffee; alcohol; oils; roasted nuts and seeds; and herbs such as cilantro.

Earth: sweet root and ground vegetables cooked into a soup, stew or casserole; stewed fruits; apple juice; and honey.

Metal: baked, pressure-cooked, or long-cooked grains such as brown rice, wheat, rye, barley, oats, or spelt; vegetables pickled over a long time, including *takuan* (a kind of daikon pickle).

Water: sea vegetable and other salads; raw fruit; miso and bean soups; miso (in other applications), shoyu, and sea salt; drinks and calming teas.

So, for example, to increase the presence of rising wood energy, I might eat more steamed green vegetables; to experience more fire energy, I could eat more fried foods and include onions, garlic, and ginger in the dish. To feel more earth energy I can experiment with more pumpkin and carrot soups, and have stewed apples for desert. To increase the presence of metal energy I might try some long-cooked brown rice, barley, and wheat. When I want to experience more water energy I can eat more salads, fruits, miso soups, and bean stews along with more drinks and teas.

Similarly, I could reduce my exposure to the five-element energy that is in excess by eating less of any foods associated with that element. If I felt too withdrawn, fewer metal energy foods and more fire energy foods could help. This would suggest less grain and more spicy fried vegetables. If I wanted to develop my inner strength, I could experiment with the opposite and eat slightly more grains and less fried food.

FACE READING

The five elements can be read in our faces, providing clues to the type of energy inside. In China and Japan, the five elements have been used in terms of face reading for both making a character reading and a five-element health reading.

A person with a tall forehead, a strong jaw, arching eyebrows, and ears set higher on the head or with the upper portion more developed is said to naturally have slightly more wood energy. Someone with a reddish complexion may have more fiery, midday, summer energy. Such a person may have large sparkly eyes, full cheeks, full lips, and a round, expressive face. Characteristics that describe a face with more earth energy are long, flat eyebrows possibly turning down at the ends; a broad mouth; a wider face; and ears set lower on the head. Metal energy can show up in delicate features, a bony face, thinner lips, a smaller nose, and prominent upper cheekbones. A person with more water energy might have slightly translucent skin, larger ears, a well-defined philtrum, and a more prominent chin.

A study of five-element face reading can help our understanding of the five elements in a human beings, and help us see how the five elements work in terms of human energy. Essentially, we are looking to see whether someone feels as though he or she has a spring, summer, late summer, autumn, or winter face. We can then test our reading by seeing if the person also seems to have a character that matches the season of his or her face.

FENG SHUI

The five elements form an important part of feng shui thinking. Just as each element is association with a time of year and day, it is also possible to link each five-element energy with a direction. Since wood energy describes the feeling of the sun rising in the east, we can also add the direction of the east to our list of items associated with wood energy. In this way fire is associated with the south and the midday sun, earth with the southwest and the afternoon sun, metal with the west and the sunset, and water with the north.

Once this connection is made, it becomes easy to see how different parts of a home could contain more of a certain five-element energy. For example, the east side of a building will be energized by the rising sun each morning and therefore will often have more of a wood-energy atmosphere. Spending more time there can help you absorb more wood energy.

We could also increase a five-element energy in a whole part of our home using colors, materials, and various features. For example, if we want to give a room more of a wood, spring, morning feel, we could try using a shade of green that reminds us of new springtime shoots, along with lighter, upward-moving materials such as wood; we could also emphasize upward movement with tall objects. To create a summer, midday, fire atmosphere, we could use bright reds, oranges, and purples. Beige, brown, and yellow might create an earthy, late summer, afternoon feeling. Pinks, grays, maroons, and silver could contribute to a more autumnal, sunset atmosphere. Black, white, and cream colors might create more of the winter, nighttime energy of the north.

ASTROLOGY

The five elements make up a strong component of two types of astrology: four pillar astrology and nine ki astrology. In four pillar astrology, the hour, day, month, and year of birth are looked at in terms of five-element energy and used to see if there are astrological excesses or deficiencies in any of the elements. Nine ki astrology consists of nine types of energy; each of these are recognized as having more of a particular five-element energy.

Both of these systems can sometimes lead to interesting insights that, if correct, can then be used to generate ideas regarding food, feng shui, shiatsu, qi gong, acupuncture, and other aspects of Chinese and Japanese healing arts.

SHIATSU

Shiatsu practitioners use acupressure-point diagnosis and meridian diagnosis to detect imbalances in energy, and then try to correct them through stimulating or calming the chi flowing through each meridian.

As the five elements are essentially a reflection of the daily and seasonal cycles in nature, they can be helpful in shiatsu to observing the natural energetic cycles. Pains or emotions that surface at certain times each day can be explored in terms of the five-element daily cycle, giving more clues as to a possible energetic disturbance. For example, headaches in the morning could indicate an imbalance of wood energy. Feeling stressed in the middle of the day could mean an excess of fire energy. Tiredness during the afternoon might signal poor flow of earth energy. Stiffness or tension in the evening could mean too much metal energy. Poor sleep could indicate a disturbance in water energy.

HEALING

These are some generalized examples of issues than might in theory occur if you had an excess of one of the five-element energies. You can experiment by reducing your exposure to the foods associated with that element, and increasing things associated with the other energies. You might intuitively feel that one kind of five-element energy would be particularly helpful. For example, after a period of stress you might feel drawn to the calming, cool, wintry, nighttime energy of water, while wanting to reduce fire energy.

Wood: headaches, tension, irritability, anger, a headstrong impulse. Fire: heart-related issues, high blood pressure, stress, a quick temper. Earth: sluggishness, a stuck feeling, laziness, caution. Metal: constipation, stiffness, shortness of breath, poor circulation, depression. Water: Water retention, lack of direction, a cold feeling, loneliness.

CHAPTER THIRTY-SIX

The History of Macrobiotics

To understand macrobiotics, it helps to be familiar with its history. Through researching the history of macrobiotics, you can understand the depth and breadth of the subject and get to know its key influences. For me, it's clear that macrobiotics is not about any one person or one particular interpretation.

There are two strands to macrobiotic history. One is western and the other eastern. These ran in parallel for over two thousand years until they began to be united by George Ohsawa, initially under the name of Zen macrobiotics. Michio Kushi and others took this work further, helping to create a more holistic movement.

EUROPEAN INFLUENCES

Hippocrates

The Greek physician Hippocrates (circa 460–370 BC) is famous for saying, "Let food be thy medicine and medicine thy food." This statement could be claimed to mark the beginning of macrobiotics and the study of our relationship with food. Although Hippocrates did not use the word "macrobiotics," the words "macro" and "bios" were used together in Greek philosophy to describe living a long life.

Leonardo da Vinci

Leonardo da Vinci was born in 1452 and went on to become a revolutionary painter, scientist, engineer, inventor, philosopher, and architect. He greatly furthered human understanding of anatomy, and his writing is revered among esoteric healers. Here are some of Leonardo da Vinci's thoughts on health.

"If you would keep healthy, follow this regimen: do not eat unless you feel inclined, and drink lightly; chew well, and let what you take be well cooked and simple. He who takes medicine does himself harm; do not give way to anger and avoid close air; hold yourself upright when you rise from the table." He became a vegetarian and advised moderation. He wrote, "May sobriety, healthy food and good sleep keep you in good health."

Da Vinci also wrote about love, stating, "Only love can stop hate," and, "Love overcomes all obstacles." He had some profound thoughts on life, including, "He who does not value life does not deserve it" and "While I thought I was learning how to live, I have been learning how to die." About the soul, da Vinci wrote, "For so much more worthy as the soul is than the body, so much more noble are the possessions of the soul than those of the body."

Sir Francis Bacon

In 1620, Sir Francis Bacon drew on the work of Greek philosophers to write his study of humans and nature. He started with an interesting premise: that we should clear the mind of all beliefs before developing our own understandings and philosophies.

Bacon wrote an essay called "The History of Life and Death," which explored longevity. In fact, his entire Great Instauration is about the great way of life. "Curing diseases is effected by temporary medicines; but lengthening of life requireth observation of diets," he wrote in *Of the Prolongation of Life*.

Nicholas Culpeper

Around the same time (in 1652 and 1653), English botanist Nicholas Culpeper published two books in which, to use his words, he "took a voyage to visit my mother nature" and wrote in great detail about the influence of herbs on human health. Culpeper questioned the medical practices of the time, and wanted to make medicine accessible to everyone through his books. It has been a consistent theme of macrobiotics that students and practitioners have been encouraged to take responsibility for their own health. We still have the intention to educate people to treat themselves rather than to prescribe anything, such as a diet.

Christoph Wilhelm Hufeland

German physician Christoph Wilhelm Hufeland, in his book *Makrobiotik, The*

Art of Prolonging Life, first used the word "macrobiotics" in the context of food and health in 1797. Hufeland was an influential doctor who was active in medical research and became a medical professor at Jena and, later, the first dean of medicine at the University of Berlin. He lived in the Age of Reason and, despite the title of his book, he also considered macrobiotics a science aimed at prolonging and perfecting life. According to Hufeland, macrobiotics is a medical philosophy that is on a higher level than the curative, preventative, or health levels of medicine. "The medical art must consider every disease as an evil which cannot be too soon expelled; the macrobiotic, on the other hand, shows that many diseases may be the means of prolonging life."

In his book Hufeland refers to a life force that he claimed is present in everything and most easily detected in organic beings, where it manifests in its response to external stimuli. This force can be weakened, as well as strengthened, through external influences. He believed that our life force would be depleted through physical exertion and increased with rest. Hufeland proposed that moral and physical health are intertwined and flow from the same source, both marked by an abundance of life force. In his view, illness was to be prevented primarily by pursuing a proper diet and lifestyle. In terms of using the word "macrobiotics" in relation to health, food, and energy or life force, Hufeland could be considered the founder of macrobiotics.

Charles Darwin

In 1859, Charles Darwin published his work *On The Origin of Species,* in which he presented his theories on natural selection and evolution. Darwin's ideas suggested that humankind would adapt and learn to survive in the natural environment through an abundance of reproduction and natural selection, passing evolutionary developments on to offspring. This implies that we have evolved over many generations to best succeed eating indigenous foods in season. It also suggests that local foods and eating patterns would over time come to partially define the humans who lived in a certain area. These are both common themes in macrobiotic thinking.

Furthermore, Darwin's work suggests that we evolve in the way we do for a reason, and that humans have evolved to experience anger, fear, jealousy, depression, and stress to help their own survival and the survival of the human race, even if these emotions may now hinder us in our modern lifestyles.

Helena Blavatsky

Helena Blavatsky, also known as Madame Blavatsky, cofounded the Theosophical Society in September 1875. She wrote that all religions were true in their inner teachings but also imperfect in their external, conventional manifestations. Her writings connecting esoteric spiritual knowledge with the new sciences of the time can be considered to be the beginning of what is now called new age thinking. She wrote of the ability we have to know God through our intuition.

Alice Bailey

Alice Bailey became influential in the Theosophical Society and claimed she channeled messages from the Taoist master Djwal Khul. She went on to write twenty-four books between 1919 and 1949 and through her writing she started the esoteric healing movement. She devoted much of her writing to encouraging readers to connect with their souls and live through a divine connection to the universe. Her main contribution to our practice of macrobiotics is the aim of developing and trusting our intuition.

Annie Besant

Annie Besant was a vegetarian and activist for social and women's rights. She was friends with George Bernard Shaw and later joined the Theosophical Society. This quote expresses her feelings about personal truth: "That one loyalty to Truth I must keep stainless, whatever friendships fail me or human ties be broken. She may lead me into the wilderness, yet I must follow her."

CHINESE INFLUENCES

The Yellow Emperor

The first writing on classical Chinese medicine is *The Yellow Emperor's Classic of Internal Medicine* (written sometime between 2600 BC and 200 BC), in which an understanding of the human energetic body is clearly described in terms of acupressure points and meridians of energy. The book is taken from conversations between the Yellow Emperor and his physician, and includes descriptions of yin and yang along with the five elements. The five elements are used to describe the energy of foods in terms of five kinds of tastes.

Yin and yang and the five elements are still the main principles used for developing an understanding of the connection between food, energy, and human health in macrobiotics.

Lao Tzu

Around the same period (circa 600–300 BC) the *Tao Te Ching* was written by Lao Tzu; it is often considered the most influential Taoist text. Essential themes expressed are naturalness, vitality, peace, non-action, emptiness, detachment, the strength of softness, flexibility, receptiveness, and spontaneity. This describes a way of living and being that can lead to longevity and good health. Later, aspects of this philosophy would find its way into macrobiotic thinking.

INDIAN INFLUENCES

Buddha

The roots of Buddhism can be traced back to northeastern India around 563 BC, when Siddhartha Gautama found compassion in human suffering, left his palace, and renounced materialism. He became known as Buddha (the enlightened one), and his teachings became known as Buddhism.

A cornerstone of Buddhism is a set of principles known as the Four Noble Truths: Life means suffering, as humans and the world we live in are imperfect. All suffering is caused by ignorance of nature and reality, along with the resultant attachment to transient things. Suffering can be healed by overcoming attachment to the material world. The path that leads away from suffering is the Noble Eightfold Path, consisting of correct views, intention, speech, action, livelihood, effort, mindedness, and contemplation.

The essence of this is to differentiate between reality and delusions. Basing our happiness on material wealth leads to unhappiness, and true happiness comes from inside by living in the real world. This also became a theme of macrobiotic philosophy.

Chakras

Around a similar time and perhaps earlier, the energetic body was being described in terms of seven energy centers called chakras. These are located at the top of the head, lower forehead, throat, mid-chest, solar plexus, navel, and pubic bone. Each are considered to be a center of energy that is associated with a certain aspect of the human being. These associations are open to interpretation. The terms commonly used in macrobiotic teaching are spirituality, intellect, communication, emotions, physical will, vitality, and reproduction, staring at the top of the head and working down to the pubic bone.

The chakras are often used in macrobiotic thinking to help understand connections between human energy, emotions, and thinking. The central heart chakra is commonly used as the focus for healing.

JAPANESE INFLUENCES

Eisai

In the late twelfth century, the Japanese monk Eisai sailed to China to learn more from the Ch'an masters who moved Buddhism away from scriptures to meditation; on his return to Japan, Eisai promoted the Chinese style of Zen Buddhism.

Dogen

Eisai's student Dogen returned from China to Japan around 1227 and is known for his oneness of practice-enlightenment. His writing included *Instructions for the Cook*. Dogen claimed: "To learn the Buddhist way is to learn about oneself. To learn about oneself is to forget oneself. To forget oneself is to perceive oneself as all things. To realize this is to cast off the body and mind of self and others. When you have reached this stage you will be detached even from enlightenment but will practice it continually without thinking about it."

Sen no Rikyu

The Japanese tea ceremony was established and developed in Japan in the early

1200s, and by the early 1500s it was the most recognizable expression of Zen philosophy. The Zen monk Sen no Rikyu refined the tea ceremony so that it became a means to meditation; in the process he founded the philosophy of *wabi sabi.* The key thoughts in *wabi sabi* are that nothing is perfect, everything changes, appreciation leads to a love of everything, being humble helps us explore further, embracing simplicity avoids needless distractions, developing intuition releases us from dogma, non-attachment gives us emotional freedom, tranquility nourishes the soul, living in the moment keeps us in reality, and living naturally helps us be our true selves. These are ideas that later contributed to George Ohsawa's macrobiotic philosophy.

Sagen Ishizuka

In the late 1800s, Japanese military doctor Sagen Ishizuka had great success in helping people recover from the serious health problems of the time. He carried out many clinical trials and published two large volumes of his works. His theory was that a natural diet, in which foods are eaten in season and attention is paid to the correct balance of potassium and sodium and acid and alkaline, leads to good health.

Lima and George Ohsawa

George Ohsawa recovered from tuberculosis of the lung and colon in 1911 using a diet recommended by Dr. Sagen Ishizuka. Ohsawa was so grateful for his new lease on life that he dedicated the rest of his life to continuing Dr. Ishizuka's work. He used the word "macrobiotic," joining the Greek words *macro,* meaning great, and *bios,* meaning life. His intention was to create a diet and philosophy to help people live a great life, to live life to the fullest. There are conflicting opinions as to whether he had read Christoph Wilhelm Hufeland's work, which had been translated into Japanese, and, if so, to what extent this influenced him.

Perhaps as a result of his near-death experience, Ohsawa put a huge emphasis on appreciation. From his writings, it is clear that he felt life was precious and had little patience with those who did not fully engage in life or treat their bodies with respect. Ohsawa wrote nearly three hundred books and pamphlets during his lifetime. Reading George Ohsawa's many books, you will recognize aspects of Taoist, Zen Buddhist and *wabi sabi* thinking. One of Ohsawa's most popular books is *Zen Macrobiotics.*

Key elements of Ohsawa's thinking are non belief (often written in Latin as non-credo), resisting judgments, not thinking in dualistic ways, recognizing that everything has two sides, recognizing that everything changes, self-responsibility, not being arrogant (not allowing our ego to take over), being humble, and recognizing that we can ultimately experience a oneness with our universe.

The idea that each of us is responsible for our own lives and health was a radical and pioneering thought. People tended to just live their lives, and when they were ill went to a doctor for treatment. There was little consideration given to diet.

George Ohsawa wrote and taught extensively on oneness, gratitude, appreciation, freedom, and justice. These can all be explored further by reading *Essential Ohsawa.* He also developed models in which he described seven conditions of health, sickness, and judgment. In addition, he wrote what he considered to be seven principles and twelve theorems that describe our universe.

George Ohsawa brought the principles of yin and yang into macrobiotics and described seeing the world in terms of yin and yang as wearing magic spectacles. In the process, he changed the interpretation of yin and yang from the current Chinese version to one similar to the older Fu Hsi's pre-heavens sequence.

Lima Ohsawa was George Ohsawa's wife; she taught numerous macrobiotic cooking classes, wrote a macrobiotic cookbook called *Art of Just Cooking,* and was sought after for her palm healing as described in *Practical Guide to Far Eastern Macrobiotic Medicine.*

George Ohsawa traveled extensively, spreading his message wherever he went. He ran courses on macrobiotics and trained a group of students in Japan to go out into the world and spread macrobiotics to other continents. Of these, Michio and Aveline Kushi, Herman and Cornelia Aihara, and Shizuko Yamamoto, among others, moved to North America. Tomio Kikuchi went to Brazil, where he mixed macrobiotics with martial arts and physical fitness.

Kikuchi focused on the ideas of balance and showing that we cannot have peace without something of the opposite. Madame Rivière moved to France and started activities there. Another Ohsawa student, Masahiro Oki, started the Okido yoga movement.

All these students wrote books, gave numerous lectures, and helped thousands of people explore macrobiotics. It is a great testament to George Ohsawa's work that his students would prove to have such profound influence.

MIDDLE EASTERN INFLUENCES

Jesus

Michio Kushi used the Gospel of Thomas as a study of Jesus's teachings and example of his relevance to our exploration of macrobiotics and life. This quote helps us put food into perspective: "If you go into any land and walk about in the regions, if they receive you, eat what is set before you; heal the sick among them. For what goes into your mouth will not defile you; but what comes out of your mouth, that is what will defile you."

This teaching can be read as an instruction in not being dualistic in our thinking, not separating reality from our thoughts, or, simply, in being holistic: "When you make the two one, you will become sons of man, and when you say: Mountain, move away, it will move away."

Here, Jesus can be said to be talking about asking questions, exploring, enjoying the process, and searching, rather than wanting answers or results: "Since you have discovered the beginning, why do you seek the end? For where the beginning is, there will the end be. Blessed is he who shall stand at the beginning, and he shall know the end, and shall not taste death."

MODERN INFLUENCES

Michio and Aveline Kushi

With the help of Michio and Aveline Kushi, macrobiotic centers and communities sprouted up throughout America and Europe during the late 1970s;

these communities became the place to go if you wanted to learn about energy, yin and yang, the five elements, trigrams, and karma. During this time there was a huge explosion of interest in everything from the East. Aveline, Michio, and their colleagues were also responsible for bringing tofu, miso, sea vegetables, *umeboshi,* and bancha tea to the West. Michio brought many aspects of classical Chinese and Japanese healing into his classes.

Inevitably, many of the practices that were associated with macrobiotics in America and Europe grew up and eventually left the macrobiotic family. As time went by, even subjects like yin and yang and the five elements were no longer seen as associated with macrobiotics. Macrobiotic ideas that were pioneering in the late '70s and early '80s became mainstream in the '90s. Michio and Aveline Kushi gave macrobiotics a greater worldview and brought in more cultural and dietary influences from around the world. In addition, they showed students how the theory of yin and yang could be applied to literally anything; through this, they demonstrated how everything can ultimately be connected.

The pool of new things to bring to the West started to dry up, and this coincided with a time when more and more people came to macrobiotics to recover from serious health problems. This trend was largely fueled by Dr. Anthony Sattilaro's book *Recalled by Life,* which charted the author's recovery from cancer. This was in the 1980s, and macrobiotics took a more serious turn with the emphasis on healing. As the success of the movement grew and more people wrote books about their recovery from various forms of cancer through macrobiotics, the whole macrobiotic approach to eating became known as a cancer-cure diet.

One of the results of this was that the diet itself became more focused and clear. George Ohsawa had put the emphasis on how to choose healthy foods rather than on listing out all the recommended foods along with the different ways to prepare them. Using his immense experience in healing, Michio detailed what he described as the standard macrobiotic diet.

The popularity of macrobiotics with those recovering from serious illness meant that the diet and approach became more purist, with the focus on clean, healing foods. This tended to put off people who were looking for a general healthy lifestyle, and even gave macrobiotics the reputation of being extreme despite its being broadly in line with recommendations from the World Health Organization.

EMERGING INFLUENCES

A second generation of teachers has emerged in the U.S. and Europe, and they have helped update the dietary side of macrobiotics as well as bringing in some of the more recent work on emotions. William Tara, author of *Macrobiotics and Human Behavior* and the founder of London's East West Centre, Europe's largest center for alternative medicine and a focal point for macrobiotics that has attracted students from all over the world during the 1970s and 1980s, continues to develop the macrobiotic connection with emotions, society, and ecology. Greg Johnson has pioneered transformational work within macrobiotics through the Concord Institute in London.

Macrobiotics itself has now become more holistic, taking in its full, rich history and living up to the meaning of macrobiotics as a large life. As a result, it has become more flexible, with a greater emphasis on experiencing the relationship between food and healing rather than being a diet.

Many of the people who are currently shaping what we think of as macrobiotics appear in this book. The whole movement has moved into a more horizontal organization in which there are no obvious leaders but, instead, more of a collective of people working together.

I'd like to give a special thanks to David Kerr for reviewing and contributing to this chapter.

PART SIX
PRACTICAL ADVICE

This is where I would like to share my thirty years of experience in living with various macrobiotic ideas. During that time I've been a student of macrobiotics, brought up four boys, taught macrobiotic ideas, cooked macrobiotic meals, run macrobiotic centers, written books, hosted a large Internet support and discussion group, and shared experiences with numerous macrobiotic teachers and cooks.

I would claim that many people don't try macrobiotics because they think that the cooking will take too long and they feel they won't be able to give up their favorite foods. While both of those concerns would have been valid during the 1980s and 1990s, macrobiotics has evolved to become broader, easier, and more convenient. To illustrate this, we will explore the issues of shortcuts, eating out, and cravings.

Many people come to the health food shop that Dragana and I own because they are concerned about not harming their children with processed foods. One of the attractions of macrobiotics is that there is the knowledge and experience to bring up our children on healthy foods and, in theory, give them the best biological start in life. In this section I will explain how to adapt macrobiotic ideas about food for babies and children.

CHAPTER THIRTY-SEVEN
Cravings

There tend to be three types of craving: those that come about from some kind of physical need, those that result from emotional associations we have with certain foods, and those that stem from habits.

Physical cravings can come about from an imbalance in our diets. Our bodies have an amazing capacity to guide us to the foods we most need. It is partly through this mechanism that we can intuitively know what to eat. We have stored information on all the meals we have eaten and can subconsciously correlate the smells, tastes, and textures with the way we feel after eating certain foods.

All of us will get messages about imbalances in the form of cravings. Too many sodium-rich foods can result in cravings for more potassium-rich foods. Sugary foods, which precipitate the overproduction of insulin and therefore a sugar low, will result in craving for more carbohydrates to bring blood sugar levels up again. These kinds of cravings are important, as they help us work out what we might be missing and what to eat more of.

If the food we crave isn't something we want, we can look for another food with similar nutritional and energetic qualities. For example, we could substitute tahini for butter, or fried tofu for cheese; we could try chewing our grains more to break down the carbohydrates instead of consuming sugar. Each of these can satisfy our cravings on a nutritional level. We are less likely to get physical cravings if we eat a wide variety of foods prepared using a range of cooking styles. Most physical cravings come from eating a narrow, restrictive diet.

If your diet becomes too sodium-rich, you will often get cravings for more liquids, fruits, and desserts as your body tries to maintain its proper balance. If you are trying to lose weight or maintain stable blood sugar levels by avoiding foods with high sugar content, it's important to keep sodium-rich foods to a minimum. From a macrobiotic perspective, foods that are sodium-rich, high in GI and GL, and dry—such as bread, chips, crackers, or oatcakes—will precipitate strong cravings. Some chefs will mask poor-quality ingredients by adding excess salt. You could consume as much as several days worth of salt in one meal at a restaurant. Be aware of any cravings after a restaurant meal so you can learn which restaurants serve foods that are most likely to lead to cravings.

Emotional cravings come from eating certain foods and experiencing certain emotions with them over the long term. For example, if you were given ice cream as a reward or treat you when you were a child, you might find you can relive those happy emotions simply by eating ice cream. This becomes self-perpetuating, as every time you eat ice cream you will relive those feelings, increasing the strength of the association. The easiest way to combat this is to make sure that you create a happy environment whenever you eat healthy foods. Put on your favorite music, watch a DVD that makes you laugh, eat with people whose company you enjoy, place fresh flowers on the table—do whatever it takes to really feel good while you're eating your macrobiotic foods.

As time goes by, you will slowly create positive associations with your new foods. This will reach a point where the thought of miso soup, salads, cooked grains, or a bean dish is enough to give you an emotional lift.

Habitual cravings come about from getting used to, say, always having coffee and cookies at eleven in the morning or eating chocolate after dinner. We might get into the habit of going into that certain café on the way to work.

These habits and associations reside in our heads, so one way of getting out of habits is to meditate and move from our head to our heart when it's the time when we usually have our habitual foods. We can also create new, healthier habits by substituting foods that help us feel better.

Moving from our heads to our hearts can often be enough for us to realize that a craving is just an old habit or a desire for a feeling from our past, and not a meaningful craving for our current situation.

As time goes by, you may experience intuitive messages to eat certain dishes without any obvious reason. The idea is that if we can connect with our souls and remain in a receptive state, we can receive messages that will lead us to new foods that will fulfill a particular need.

CHAPTER THIRTY-EIGHT
Eating Out

Eating in restaurants and cafés can be a fun, social, and satisfying way to enjoy our food. Eating out from time to time can be part of a healthy modern lifestyle, and help bring variety to our eating habits. Going on vacation is a good opportunity to take a break from our regular foods and explore new dishes. This can be educational when visiting other countries and trying their traditional cuisines.

As there is now so much more choice when eating out, it's easier to find healthy foods. Most towns will have somewhere you can get pasta with a simple sauce and salad. By searching around, you'll find that you can eat healthily wherever you are. If there's nothing on the menu that seems right for you, try asking for your choice of pasta and salad. If you're lucky enough to find an organic restaurant, you can be assured of better-quality ingredients.

Because so many people suffer from allergies, restaurants have become more accommodating to special diets; if you are experimenting by only eating certain foods for a while, you can see if they will make dishes especially for you. In this situation, the simpler the better. For example, ask for pasta with garlic and olive oil, plain blanched broccoli, or carrots and a green salad. If in doubt, ask for any sauces or dressings to be on the side.

There are some areas of concern, and these are oils, salt, and additives; it's worth asking about these when you visit a restaurant. Most restaurants will not use expensive oils for deep frying, as they use a lot of oil. Cheap oils tend to be made from a blend of polyunsaturated oils and may break down under the extreme heat used for frying; when this happens, oils become unstable. Eating oils in this state risks introducing free radicals into your body. This can cause oxidization and accelerate the aging process. As you'll consume relatively large amounts of oil when eating deep fried foods like French fries, the risks are also higher. I tend to avoid fried or oily foods when eating out. Olive oil is ideal, but often too expensive for restaurant use. Check with the chef to see what oil a restaurant is using.

Be aware that some dishes may contain excessive quantities of salt; as a result, you might feel different for a while and require more water, salads, and fruit to return to your optimum state.

Monosodium glutamate (MSG) is often used in Chinese restaurants. You may be able to preorder dishes without MSG, or there may be certain dishes that don't have it. If you don't wish to eat meat, ask about soup stocks, as these may contain animal products.

When eating out, my family's favorite restaurants are Japanese, Italian, and Indian; I have also often enjoyed eating Greek, French, and Chinese foods. We like to eat quite widely when going out, knowing that it's not everyday food and that it can be helpful to expand and alter our normal repertoire. Here are some examples of foods to try when going out, and tips on healthy restaurant eating.

Pasta with pesto, vegetable, or seafood sauce.

Vegetable soup with a good-quality bread.

Salads.

Vegetables cooked al dente without butter, if you want that fresh, clean taste.

Pita bread with hummus, tahini, falafel, and salad.

Noodles in a hot broth; however, check to see if they use MSG in the broth. Broth can also be very salty, in which case do not drink it.

Sushi. The white rice will often have some sugar in it. If you want to avoid the rice, ask for sashimi. Japanese restaurants often have an interesting variety of vegetable dishes, sea vegetable salads, tofu dishes, and pickles, along with items that include natto.

Try natto maki (natto in a sushi roll), natto oroshi (natto, grated daikon and mushrooms), or natto yamakake (natto, a grated mountain potato, and raw tuna).

Fish and seafood dishes. Fish soups tend to be particularly high in nutrients. Try young herring for a high mineral content. The cleanest will be a poached white fish with lemon. The best fish will be those that are most fresh. In that case there is little need to dress the fish up and coat it with rich sauces.

Lentil and vegetable curries. Sometimes the chef will add a lot of oil; however, as liquid-based dishes like curry cannot reach a temperature higher than the boiling point, there is less risk of the oil breaking down.

Basmati rice is more nutritious and has a lower GI than white rice.

A good-quality pizza. If you do not want a lot of cheese, try focaccia, bruschetta, or a pizza without cheese.

Naan bread can be very satisfying and less bloating than highly yeasted breads.

In cafés my family and I might eat croissants, scones, cakes, and pastries. We also like a rich dessert from time to time; this can be anything, including tiramisu, profiteroles, cheesecake, or apple strudel, as well as my mother's trifle, meringues, or delicious apple pies. I usually drink herbal teas when out, but sometimes I enjoy a very mild coffee. When possible I like to drink fresh vegetable or fruit juices. A smoothie can also be refreshing.

CHAPTER THIRTY-NINE
Quick Meals

If our aim with macrobiotics is to live the big life, spending too much time in the kitchen doesn't allow us to get out and make the most of ourselves. It is therefore helpful to practice macrobiotics in such a way that you get the right balance between eating homemade, natural, healthy foods and having the time to develop yourself.

When I started practicing macrobiotics, it was typical to spend at least an hour or two cooking a meal. Since then I have learned how to organize myself better so that I cook time-consuming dishes only once every three days, meaning that the remaining days' meals are quick and easy.

EASIER THAN YOU THINK

Macrobiotic cooking is very easy. Essentially, all we do is heat up water and put ingredients in. Sometimes we leave the ingredients in to make a soup or stew, and sometimes we take them out again. For most recipes, it's as simple as that. Frying can require more attention. Baking can require experience and skill.

I would suggest that the most important piece of equipment for macrobiotic cooking is a timer. The dishes that take the longest to cook—for example, brown rice, bean soups, and stews—require very little attention. Once they are simmering away, I get on with something else and wait for my timer to let me know when to turn off the heat.

Planning Ahead

I find it helps to plan ahead so that I have soaked or precooked ingredients ready for certain meals. For example, soaking some grains or beans before I go to bed means everything is ready for me the next day. Cooking extra brown rice and barley in the evening will mean I have leftovers to make a porridge in the morning, to fry for lunch, or for Dragana to make a rice pudding in the evening. Similarly, when I want to eat a whole oat porridge, I cook enough whole oats for a week and then warm up a bowlful each morning.

Keeping the Essentials in Your Kitchen

When you want to eat more healthily, it's important to always have a stock of healthy foods in your refrigerator and cupboards. This way you can quickly create a healthy meal rather than be tempted to reach for a less healthy snack. For this to work, it's helpful to have a bowl of a cooked whole grain, some cooked beans, and pot of soup in your fridge so all you need to do is heat them up to make a meal.

In addition, keep all the ingredients to make quick ten-minute meals, so you can come home feeling hungry knowing that within ten minutes you will be eating a healthy macrobiotic meal.

Every Third Day

I can eat a healthy macrobiotic diet using predominantly whole, living foods every day, but it's only every third day that I spend more than twenty minutes in the kitchen. On each third day I may spend one and a half hours getting everything ready for a meal.

On my big cooking day, I make a big pot of whole grains; if I don't include beans with the grains, I cook a bean stew or soup. I will also make some longer-cooked vegetables in the form of a stew or thick soup. I try to estimate how much to cook to last until my next big cooking day. For example, two cups of a whole grain can make enough for four people to eat dinner, lunch, and dinner again, depending on everyone's appetite. You will need to store cooked foods in a fridge to make them last. With leftovers, it's very important to heat up only the food you are going to eat rather than heating the all the food, as cooling and heating shortens the life of food and can increase the risk of growing harmful bacteria.

You can take your leftover grains and fry them, steam them to heat them up, cook them into a soup or boil them into a soft porridge to make them more interesting. To make these meals complete, I would add light fresh dishes such as a pressed salad or blanched or steamed vegetables.

On other days I'll use millet or corn if I want a quick-cooking whole grain, or mochi, noodles, couscous, or pasta if I want a processed grain. I will lightly boil or steam vegetables to go with the grain, make a salad, and add some pickles. For greater richness I might fry some tofu. Once you are familiar with the recipes, these meals are very quick to make.

It's important to be able to make quick, healthy macrobiotic meals so that you aren't in a position where you feel you cannot eat the way you want because you don't have enough time. In fact, it's often just as quick and easy to make a healthy meal as a less healthy one. It just requires a little time to become familiar with the ingredients and learn how to prepare them.

There are now plenty of readily available ingredients that will allow you to make a healthy macrobiotic meal quickly. For example, mochi, tofu, natto, vegetable burgers (or those made with beans or grains), natural pesto sauces, natural sauerkraut, good-quality breads, hummus, tahini, organic canned beans, natural live yogurt, and stewed fruit can all be bought readymade and need very little or no preparation.

There are some foods that are generally better to make yourself, such as miso soup, whole grains, and sauces; the instant varieties do not have the living energy of freshly made versions, or similar levels of nutrition.

Here are some examples of quick macrobiotic meals that you can make without any precooked foods.

Breakfast: miso soup; fried mochi seasoned with maple syrup, honey, or shoyu and brown rice vinegar; steamed bread with hummus and sauerkraut; polenta with yogurt and sunflower seeds; organic muesli with rice, oat, or nut milk. Pair any of these with vegetable juice and/or herb tea.

Lunch or dinner: corn on the cob, tuna, and vegetables; vegetables and potato salad; couscous and vegetables; noodles and vegetables; fried mochi and vegetables. Pair any of these with miso soup and fresh salad and/or fresh fruit.

If you are following the shortcuts principle, you may already have precooked foods available. If this is the case, you can do the following to make meals quickly.

Breakfast: Heat up leftover whole oat porridge.

Lunch or Dinner: heat up any leftover soup; use leftover grains steamed, fried, put into a soup, or at room temperature; steam or fry leftover millet; heat up barley stew. Pair any of these with fresh steamed, blanched, or raw vegetables, pickles, and/or fried fish.

Note: When reheating foods it's important to heat up only the amount of food you're going to eat and to make sure it's heated all the way through. Failure to do this can result in the growth of potentially harmful bacteria. The aim is to reheat the foods in a way that all the food reaches a temperature of at least seventy degrees centigrade (158 degrees Fahrenheit). This temperature is too high for the bacteria to survive. Make sure you stir any thick soups so all the liquid reaches the boiling point; when frying leftover grains, fry a thin layer and turn frequently. To steam leftovers, use small amounts and break up any clumps of food so that the center is exposed to the steam; when boiling leftovers, allow sufficient time for the heat to reach the center of foods. The larger the piece of food, the longer it will take.

CHAPTER FORTY
Babies and Children

The macrobiotic community has a wealth of experience of bringing up children. There have been many successes and quite few challenges. Through our collective learning we have accumulated some interesting observations.

I have experienced raising four boys, and I've shared my experiences with those of my sister, Melanie, who has raised seven children and helped many mothers over the years.

The experiences I would like to share here are about feeding babies and children, as well as some about bringing up children in general. I stress that these are generalizations based on my experience; your child is unique and may require a different approach. My intention is to give you some broad suggestions to try out and play with so that you can experience a range of options and see which works best for you and your child.

FEEDING BABIES

Ideally, you will initially start by breast-feeding your child so that he or she can benefit from the complete nutrition your milk provides and also form a strong emotional and energetic bond with you. There are no rules for how long to breast-feed. Some mothers will breast-feed for six months and start introducing other foods slowly; others will wait. I have known mothers who continue to breast-feed until their children are three years old while also feeding the children solid foods as well.

Much will depend on the needs of your child and how much milk you can provide. There's no right or wrong here, and what to do it will become clear from trusting in your own intuition and sharing your experiences with other mothers. I would caution you against trying to follow some conceptual idea on how long to breast-feed, or to try to serve your own needs through extending breast-feeding when deep down you are aware it is not best for your child.

Some women become tired and eventually exhausted from long-term breast feeding. Try to find those moments when you can meditate and be in your heart so you can feel what would be best for you and your baby.

When you feel your baby is ready to start with other foods you can try some homemade grain milk, fruit juice, puréed vegetables, stewed fruit, or any combination of these. Certain foods, such as beans, cauliflower, onions, cabbage, and broccoli, can increase wind. It is generally recommended you don't add any salt to your child's food until he or she is at least two. At this stage you have the opportunity to help your child get used to other tastes and develop his or her digestive system to absorb a wider range of foods. While you are still breast-feeding, your child will benefit from a wide range of nutrients.

One you stop breast-feeding, your child will require a full range of nutrients from his or her food. Although some children have enjoyed excellent health eating a range of whole foods, not all thrive on a diet devoid of animal foods and processed grains. My general advice would be to give your child a broad diet and include some fish, eggs, dairy foods, and, if you feel it's appropriate, meat; this is generally more helpful than being unnecessarily restrictive.

Some mothers cannot produce breast milk in sufficient quantity. Rich foods can encourage the production of breast milk. In macrobiotic folklore, mochi, fish soups, and dark beer are thought to aid the production of breast milk. If you still cannot produce enough milk, you will need to bring in grain milks, puréed vegetables, and other liquids early. I would also consider supplementing this with some organic sheep's, cow's, and/or goat's milk.

Grain milk can be made by cooking various whole grains in five times as much water as grain for about two hours. You may need to add even more water during cooking to keep the consistency watery and creamy. Once cooked, strain the grain through a sieve or cloth and collect the liquid in another pot. You can mix in honey, puréed vegetables, stewed fruit, ground-up roasted seeds and nuts, as well as oil, to create a sweet-tasting, rich milk.

A widely used remedy for sore nipples caused by breast-feeding is to put grated carrot over your nipples between feedings. You can keep the grated carrot in position with a cloth and bra.

FEEDING CHILDREN

I have met parents who have an artificial goal of bring their children up without any exposure to animal foods or sugar; they often seem to judge themselves on their ability to do this. There's no evidence that a child brought up like this will be healthier than a child who occasionally eats a little animal food or added sugar when at a party or eating out.

As we don't really know our children's nutritional needs, I suggest our main goal is to introduce our children to as many natural foods as possible, and help them develop sensitivity and experience-based knowledge of what foods will help them most. It may be that the biggest favor you give your children is the benefit of acquiring the taste for a wide range of generally healthy foods.

Children will naturally home in on a few foods they enjoy the taste of, develop favorites, and then tend to want to just eat those foods repeatedly. Part of our parental guidance is to encourage our children to at least keep trying other foods. In my family we tried having a rule at mealtimes that our children at least try a tiny amount of everything. Even though they didn't like many foods initially, we found that over time they acquired a taste for them and would later ask for those foods at meals.

Most children I know naturally go through a phase of loving processed grains like pasta and bread, and showing a limited interest in vegetables. This can be a trying phase for the health-conscious parent. During this phase we found that whether the vegetable was raw, steamed, blanched, or cooked for a long time made a huge difference as to whether it was eaten. With our children, overcooking the vegetable even slightly meant it was pushed to one side. I would encourage any parent to keep experimenting with different cooking styles to find those that most appeal to their children.

In addition, our children liked being able to dip their vegetables in a variety dips. Hummus, tahini, vinegar, shoyu mixed with brown rice vinegar, oils, and nut butters tended to make vegetables more appetizing to them.

A variety of fresh fruit can provide useful nutrients and be a source of natural living energy. Fruit makes an excellent snack or dessert. It can be mixed with salads to enhance the appeal for a child.

Most important is to try and encourage an association between eating healthy foods and generally feeling good. Forcing a child to eat something he or she does not like or punishing a child for not eating something will only create a negative association, and risks putting them off that food for a long time.

Denying or limiting certain foods will often make them become more appealing. For example, keeping chocolate in the house to give your child as a reward for good behavior, a special treat, or, worse, a bribe for doing something will make the chocolate feel like a highly desirable food to your child. If you really want to carry out these practices, it would make sense to at least do it with something that is potentially more healthy and less addictive, such as fruit.

One way Dragana and I tried bringing up our children was to give them access to a range of foods, including various snacks, and to let them eat these when they felt like it. This would include fruit, nuts, seeds, raisins, organic crackers, cookies, and leftover desserts. We would not keep foods like ice cream, soft drinks, or sugary snacks in the house. This way the children seemed to get used to what was available and had the freedom to eat when they felt like it. Our only rule was that they would need to be able to eat their meals. If they ate too many snacks and could not eat their meals, then we would encourage them to reduce their snacks.

When we went out with them, we would generally let them choose whatever they liked. We wanted them to feel a sense of freedom and not that we had totally imposed our ideas of healthy eating on them. So they might choose pizza, various desserts, ice cream, fruit juices, smoothies, cakes, or chocolate, depending on the situation.

As discussed earlier, an overly clean, sterile environment can be unhealthy in terms of not giving our immune systems enough exercise. Try to relax enough to let your children be exposed to small amounts of organic dirt regularly, so that their immune systems will develop the resources to deal with my serious challenges and learn when they need to react.

BRINGING UP CHILDREN

I have found babies to be particularly sensitive to human emotions and energy.

If a parent feels stressed, angry, irritable, or nervous, the child will tend to react and not be able to relax. When the parents are relaxed, having fun, laughing, kind, jovial, caring, and loving, the baby or child feels secure, relaxed, and more open. This can make a big difference during mealtimes. If you get tense, and the meals develop into something of a battle as you try to get your child to eat, this becomes a stressful, unpleasant experience for everyone; it is not conducive to stimulating the appetite or eating.

Because of babies' and children's sensitivity to energy, they often enjoy some kind of touch healing. Laying your hand on your child's back, chest, or abdomen can feel very relaxing, encouraging feelings of security and helping your child through discomfort.

It seems to be part of the natural process of growing for children to experiment with testing the boundaries of human patience, perhaps as part of developing our social sensibilities and skills. Probably the safest person to try this out on is our mothers. It can be easy to take this process personally if you are the recipient of your child's tantrums, stubbornness, or willful desire to be difficult.

One starting point for all this is to ensure that your child at least feels heard and understood. Although you might not agree or let him or her do something, it can help to acknowledge the request and carefully explain your reasoning. If you can find a way to communicate with love, humor, and a sense of empathy, some of the emotional disturbances melt away.

I like to remind myself that children are not born to fit into our complex social conventions, current assumptions on life, and value judgments. It's perfectly healthy for any child to question the absurdity of all they encounter, and I hope I have encouraged my children in this. My children have challenged many of my ideas and helped me develop and evolve as a human.

Children can be like sponges, soaking up everything around them. Without realizing it they will be soaking up the way you behave and react to different situations. Your own ways of doing things may come out when your child becomes a parent. Sometimes it is more effective to just be yourself and be the kind of self you feel will pass on the characteristics you most like about yourself.

PART SEVEN
MENU PLANS

In this section I have written four different menu plans as a rough guide to how you can play with macrobiotic ideas to bring about different biological, emotional, and energetic changes in yourself.

You may find initially it is easier to follow a diet in order to get used to the foods and experience how you can feel eating a variety of macrobiotic-style foods. This stage allows you to benefit from other people's experience and learn from their successes and mistakes.

During the next stage, you may find you can move to eating with a greater understanding and experience of your relationship to food. You might use some of the principles like acid and alkaline, the GI and GL, the living energy in foods, yin and yang, and the five elements to help explore your relationship with food in different ways and create a greater awareness of how food can influence you.

Remember that with all these sample diets you can add a full range of seasonings and herbs. Adjust the taste to suit your palette with various oils, vinegars, herbs, mild spices, garlic, ginger, chopped spring onions, nori, shoyu, miso, and *umeboshi*.

In the third stage, you will hopefully reach the point where you develop your own intuition and eat to nourish your body, heart, and soul.

CHAPTER FORTY-ONE
Getting Started

I've witnessed thousands of people start their macrobiotic journeys; this happens in many different ways. Some take an all-or-nothing approach, clearing out their kitchens and refilling them with the macrobiotic foods they want to eat. If this is your style, then you might like to start with the recovery diet in Chapter Forty-Four for a few days or weeks.

With the suggestions below, I want to show you how you can slowly change your patterns of eating one step at a time by substituting one food for another. Here are some examples.

BREAKFAST

Try oatmeal or polenta porridge instead of cereals with milk and sugar. Try whole grain toast with tahini and sugar-free jam instead of white toast with butter and sugary jam. Try herb teas instead of coffee. Try a fresh vegetable juice instead of milk.

LUNCH

Try a whole-grain bread sandwich with hummus, cucumber, and herbs instead of a cheese sandwich. Try a sandwich made from pita bread, falafel, tahini, hummus, and salad instead of a meat sandwich. Try taking a thick soup to work in a wide-mouthed thermos instead of eating French fries. When eating out, order a fish dish or bean soup and a large salad instead of processed grains. At home, try corn on the cob, vegetables, and fried tofu or fish instead of bread, pasta, or premade meals. Try taking leftovers from the previous night's dinner instead of eating a takeout lunch. Try dipping your bread in olive oil and vinegar instead of spreading on butter, margarine, or cheese. Drink a fresh vegetable juice, fruit smoothie, or fruit juice instead of a sugary soft drink or coffee.

DINNER

Try introducing a miso soup occasionally. Add more vegetable dishes so that about half your plate is taken up by vegetables. Try some form of fermented food. This could mean having a little sauerkraut, gherkins, miso, shoyu, pickles, or natto with your normal meal. Try replacing meat with fish for a while. Try replacing dairy foods with tofu, hummus, tahini, and oils for while. Try eating a whole, unprocessed grain, such as brown rice, once a week. Experiment with using honey, apple juice, raisins, maple syrup, and fruit instead of sugar to sweeten dishes. Try drinking water instead of alcohol at your meal. Try eating a fruit-based dessert such as stewed fruit, fruit salad, or fruit pie instead of a dessert that is high in sugar and fats. Try a relaxing herb tea after your meal.

SNACKS

Try fresh fruit, dried fruit, nuts, or seeds instead of cookies and chocolate. Try raw vegetables and hummus instead of sweets or cake. Try a fresh vegetable or fruit juice, or a fruit smoothie, instead of sweets or cake. Try a healthy home-made cake or snack instead of a readymade one.

I would suggest you give yourself three months to slowly change your habits around certain foods, and then, when you feel ready, try the recovery diet in Chapter Forty-Four for a week or two.

CHAPTER FORTY-TWO

Low Glycemic Index and Glycemic Load Diet

The aim of this diet is to keep your blood sugar as stable as possible. This can help you achieve more consistent energy levels, greater emotional stability, and better chemical consistency at a cellular level. You may find that while eating this way you experience fewer cravings for food, lose weight, and feel calmer.

Breakfast

whole oats or leftover whole grains made into a porridge

and / or

miso soup

herb tea

and/or

fresh vegetable juice

Lunch

salad with yogurt or fried tofu or fish

or

vegetable, bean or fish soup with pickles and vegetables

or

bean curry and vegetables

or

fried tuna or tofu and vegetables

or

a large salad

Dessert
fresh fruit

or

a fresh fruit and vegetable juice

Dinner

miso, bean, fish, or vegetable soup

Main course
brown rice mixed with barley, rye, or whole wheat with a bean stew,
vegetables, and pickles

or

fish or beans, and vegetables

or

brown basmati rice, bean curry, yogurt, and vegetables

or

potato and vegetable salad

or

barley stew and vegetable dish

Dessert
fresh fruit, a fresh vegetable and fruit juice, or a fruit smoothie

Snacks
fresh fruit; roasted nuts and seeds; raw carrots, celery, and cucumber
with hummus; rye bread with tahini, nut butter, or olive oil

CHAPTER FORTY-THREE
Alkaline-Forming Diet

The aim of this diet is to help your body become more alkaline. The emphasis will be on alkaline-forming foods. For this to work, you will need to remain calm and not let yourself feel stressed. This diet goes with meditating on your breath, laughter, stretching, light exercise, and spending time in nature.

You can use this diet for any issue that you think is stress-related. It might help with various skin conditions, digestive ailments, headaches, osteoarthritis, and general aches and pains, as well as asthma. Some people claim that being more alkaline reduces the risk of cancer, and others suggest it increases the effectiveness of our immune systems.

Breakfast

blanched, steamed, or fried vegetables
and/or
miso soup

herb tea
and/or
fresh vegetable juice

Lunch

large salad
or
vegetable soup, pickles, and vegetables
or
brown basmati rice, bean curry, and plenty of vegetables

or

corn on the cob, fried tofu, and lots of vegetables

Dessert

fresh or cooked fruit

or

fresh fruit or vegetable juice

Dinner

miso or vegetable soup

Main course

brown rice mixed with barley, rye, or whole wheat,
with bean stew, vegetables, and pickles

or

millet and vegetables

or

brown basmati rice, bean curry, yogurt, and vegetables

or

potato and vegetable salad

or

barley stew and vegetable dish

Dessert

fresh fruit, stewed fruit, fresh vegetable and fruit juice,
or a fruit smoothie

Snacks

fresh fruit, roasted almonds, or raw carrots, celery,
and cucumber with hummus

Ideally, you would test your saliva with pH sticks while trying this diet. After three or four days of eating these foods, your saliva pH readings should be between 7.0 and 7.5. Once you have achieved this for a further three days, slowly bring in other foods while testing your saliva to make sure it doesn't become acidic again. If your pH readings fall below 7.0, try eating more vegetables, drinking more fresh vegetable juices or herb teas, and being more careful not to feel stressed.

As you can see, this diet is reasonably similar to the low GI and GL diet, so you can also use it to maintain stable blood sugar levels.

CHAPTER FORTY-FOUR
Recovery Diet

Here I have suggested a diet I think of as a recovery diet. These are the kinds of foods I eat when I want to feel generally more centered, clear, and balanced. I like to eat this way for a few days simply to get back to my preferred state. Sometimes I will eat these dishes for a few weeks and, in general, they form the foundation to my overall eating.

This would be an interesting diet to try for a month once you are familiar with the recipes; it may be one you might like to come back to frequently when you feel like treating yourself to foods aimed at better health.

Eating these foods will provide you with an opportunity to try developing your awareness of food and learning more about your relationship with food. As you follow this menu plan, listen to your body, heart, and mind, and be aware of how you feel.

In this menu plan, dinner is the largest meal of the day; however, it is fine to swap the meals around if you like.

Breakfast

whole oat porridge
or
polenta porridge

herb tea
and/or
fresh vegetable juice

Lunch

bean and vegetable soup

Main Course
vegetables and salad

or

mochi, polenta, vegetables, and salad

or

corn on the cob, tuna or tofu, vegetables, and salad

or

potatoes, vegetables, and salad

or

large salad

Dessert
If desired, fresh fruit

Dinner

miso or lentil soup

Main course
millet croquettes and vegetables

or

whole grains, bean and vegetable stew, and salad

or

brown basmati rice, bean curry, yogurt, and vegetables

or

couscous and vegetables

or

noodles in broth, vegetables, and pickles

or

barley stew and vegetables

or

fish, bean sauce, salad, and vegetables

Dessert

amasake kanten (a gelled dessert made from a fermented rice drink)

or

steamed apricot with fruit sauce

or

rice pudding

Snacks

fresh fruit, roasted nuts and roasted seeds, raw carrots, celery, and cucumber with hummus, raisins, or whole grain bread with tahini and sauerkraut

PART EIGHT
RECIPES

Macrobiotics is so much more than the food we consume. By chang-ing the way we fuel our bodies, we change who we are as humans. We develop our intuition and our compassion for all things living and, suddenly, all the theories and principles that make up macrobiotics come alive and become the full expression of our souls, without the limitations we experience in our physical bodies.

Once we understand harmony and balance, we can be as individ-ual as we desire and yet remain a part of the collective one that makes humanity endlessly capable of creating and sharing love—for each other, for nature, and for the universe. Our individual personalities become the glue that binds us together to the here and now, but at the same time allows us to create and shape the future we desire.

—CHRISTINA PIRELLO, cooking teacher, TV show host,
and author of *This Crazy Vegan Life*

This section contains a range of recipes that correspond to the photographs in the color insert. Each recipe is designed for one person; so you can increase them for more people or double the quan-tities if you want leftovers for the next day. The recipes include sug-gestions for breakfast, lunch, dinner, and snacks. Please feel free to play with the recipes, experiment, and explore.

CHAPTER FORTY-FIVE

Breakfasts

These recipes are generally for one person, however, where it is just as easy to cook a greater quantity and keep extras for following meals the proportions are increased.

Please feel free to experiment and play with these recipes. Relax and let your intuition guide you to making any changes that feel good to you. Remember to eat with awareness and learn from each meal.

Whole Oat Porridge

9 ounces whole oats

45 to 63 ounces water

A handful of raisins

1 tablespoon of honey or maple syrup (optional)

1 small basket of berries

10 to 15 hazelnuts

1 sprig of mint

Make this the night before you want to eat it. Wash the oats and place them in a pot that holds at least 4 pints/2 liters. Add water to the pot and place it on the stove. Switch on the burner and bring the oats to a boil. Boil for 30 minutes. Turn off the heat and leave the pot overnight.

The oats will absorb lots of liquid overnight, so in the morning, check to make sure that there's still some water in with the oats. If not, add just enough to cover the oats. Add the raisins. Give it a stir, turn on the heat, and cook over a low flame for another 10 to 15 minutes. The longer you cook the oats, the creamier they get. Switch the heat off and leave the porridge to rest. Spoon out enough for one serving in a nice bowl. Place fruits, nuts, and sweetener on top of your porridge and garnish with mint (mint goes well with summer fruits).

Place the rest of the cooked oats in a glass or stainless steel container and refrigerate them. Each morning, take a sufficient amount for breakfast, add some extra water, and heat it up. Vary what you put on top. Here are some suggestions: pears, apples, pitches, bananas, plums, oranges, any other fruit you like, dried fruit (apricots, figs, goji berries, dates), and a variety of nuts: walnuts, almonds, pecans, brazil nuts, or others.

Seeds are a lovely addition, too.

Bancha Tea

> 1 tablespoon of bancha twigs
> 2 pints/1 liter of water

In my home, we have a kettle dedicated to bancha tea. One of the reasons for this is that you can reuse the twigs. Each time you're making fresh tea, add ½ to 1 teaspoon of fresh twigs and more water. After 2 to 3 days, discard all the twigs and start fresh. Our plants love the old bancha twigs (or you can put them on your compost pile, if you have one). Another reason for the bancha kettle is that you can keep the tea in it and drink it throughout a day, either warmed up or at room temperature, which is lovely and refreshing during warm weather.

To make the tea, place the ingredients in a pot, bring to a boil, simmer for 3 to 5 minutes, and turn it off. Let stand for several minutes, and then serve.

Different kinds of tea all come from the same bush. Kukicha or bancha twig tea, as its name says, comes from the twigs of the tea bush. When young leaves from the bush are picked in the spring, they are used in making of green tea. Bancha twig tea has less caffeine than green. It is very alkaline, and it is recommended for digestive problems caused by too much acidity. It is said to be good for babies who are teething (put your finger in a cup of tea and then rub it onto the baby's teeth and gums).

Polenta Porridge with Yogurt

  5 ounces organic polenta
  4 cups cold water
  1 tablespoon sunflower seeds
  Yogurt (to taste)

Place the polenta and water in a saucepan. Cover and bring to a boil; uncover, reduce the heat to low, put a flame deflector under the pan, and simmer for 10 to 15 minutes, stirring from time to time. Turn off the heat and take out enough for one serving. Add yogurt and sprinkle the sunflower seeds on top. If you would like your polenta to taste richer, you can roast your sunflower seeds. You will need a heavy cast-iron or stainless steel skillet. Add a few drops of olive oil—enough to coat the pan but not so much that the seeds would be swimming in it—and spread it around with pastry brush. Heat up the pan for 1 or 2 minutes; then add the sunflower seeds. Roast, stirring occasionally, for a few minutes, until the seeds are nice and brown but not burnt. To add color and flavor, add seasonal fruit of your choice and/or mint leaves.

CHAPTER FORTY-SIX

Lunches

Red Quinoa, Tofu, and Vegetable Salad with Fresh Green Herbs and Egg

1 cup of red quinoa, precooked

2 medium tomatoes, cut into small chunks

1 medium clove of garlic, very finely chopped

2 to 4 tablespoons olive oil

½ cup broccoli, cut into small florets, steamed for a minute or two

¼ teaspoon sea salt

¼ teaspoon turmeric

6 to 8 olives

1 to 2 tablespoons capers

1 tablespoon fresh oregano (or ¼ teaspoon dried)

¼ cup arame sea vegetable

4 to 5 small Italian spicy peppers (peperoncini)

3 to 4 fresh shiitake mushrooms, cut into quarters

5 ounces tofu, cut into small chunks and fried

1 small apple, cut into little cubes

A handful of fresh arugula

A few sprigs each of fresh flat-leaf parsley, basil, coriander, and mint

1 organic, free-range egg (optional)

Cook the quinoa according to the package instructions.

Soak the arame by just covering with water.

While the quinoa is cooking, mix together in a deep bowl the chopped tomatoes, garlic, 1 tablespoon olive oil, steamed broccoli, and sea salt. Leave to marinate until the quinoa is finished.

When the quinoa is done, place it in a large serving bowl and sprinkle the turmeric on top. Add the olives, capers, and chopped-up fresh oregano. Gently mix with a wooden spoon.

Cook the arame for 5 to 10 minutes in a small pot. Take it out and add it to the quinoa.

Heat a tablespoon of olive oil in a skillet and fry the peperoncini for 2 to 3 minutes. Take them out and discard (they are solely to flavor the oil and the oil will remain spicy). Gently fry the shiitake mushrooms for a minute; take them out and add them to the quinoa. Then fry the tofu pieces for a few minutes and add those to the quinoa, too. Add the apple cubes to the quinoa.

Boil the egg for 4 to 5 minutes. Take out, cool off, and peel. Cut it up in quarters or slice it.

Take a third deep bowl that can hold all the ingredients and mix the quinoa and the tomato/broccoli mixture together. Place the egg on top or on one side. On another side, place the washed arugula mixed with the parsley, basil, coriander, and mint leaves (just a few of each is enough). Watercress goes well too if you cannot find the other ingredients. Sprinkle another tablespoon of olive oil on the final mixture before eating.

Polenta, Mochi, Broccoli, and Salad Lunch

    1 tablespoon sunflower seeds
    1 cup very finely shredded white cabbage
    ¼ medium-sized onion red (or yellow) onion, finely sliced in half-moons
    1 teaspoon cold-pressed organic sunflower oil
    ¼ teaspoon sea salt
    2 tablespoons sauerkraut (naturally fermented with no sugar or preservatives
        added), drained and finely chopped
    A few olives
    2 to 3 medium broccoli florets
    ½-inch slice of daikon, finely grated (preferably using a ginger grater)

½ teaspoon unhulled tahini (sesame paste)

A few drops *umeboshi* vinegar

¼ teaspoon unpeeled fresh grated ginger

A small amount of olive oil for frying

1 ¾-inch thick slice of polenta (see Homemade Polenta, next page)

1 piece of mochi (sweet pounded brown rice),

   typically 1 inch wide and 2 inches long

Place a small pot (about 6 inches in diameter) half filled with water on the stovetop. Bring it to a boil.

Meanwhile, dry roast the sunflower seeds: Heat a cast-iron (or stainless steel) skillet, add the seeds, and gently stir the seeds for a few minutes. They should be a lovely golden color, and not brown or burnt. Take them out of the skillet and place them in a small dish. (At home we dry roast larger amounts of various seeds—pumpkin, sunflower, sesame—once a week or so and keep them in tightly sealed jars. This way they make a lovely addition to various dishes throughout the week and are very handy when you feel like snacking. They can also be eaten raw, but we find that their taste and crunchiness is enhanced when lightly roasted.)

In an attractive serving bowl, mix the cabbage and the onions. Add the sunflower oil and sea salt and mix gently with your hands for a minute or so. Add the sauerkraut and mix it in. Garnish with a few olives and then add the sunflower seeds. Place one portion on a plate. This coleslaw-style salad can be made in larger amounts and kept in the refrigerator. Each time you want to eat it, take the desired amount out of the refrigerator and leave it out to warm up to room temperature, then eat. Finely chopped fresh parsley makes a lovely addition to this dish.

When the water is boiling, add the broccoli florets, wait for a minute, without waiting for the water to reboil, and scoop them out. The broccoli should be deep green in color and have a lovely, crunchy bite to it. Place it next to the coleslaw on your plate.

Mix the daikon with the tahini and 5 to 6 drops of *umeboshi* vinegar. Put the grated ginger on top.

Heat just enough olive oil to cover in a cast-iron skillet (you can use a brush). When the oil is hot, add the mochi and the polenta. Cover and cook for about 2 to 3 minutes on a medium flame. Turn the mochi and polenta over and cook for another 2 minutes. Remove and place on a plate. You can, if you wish, season the mochi with a drop or two of shoyu and a drop or two of brown rice or apple cider vinegar.

Add the polenta and mochi to the plate, and serve with the daikon mixture on top.

Homemade Polenta

If you can't buy premade polenta (which these days is available in supermarkets), this is how you make your own.

> 1½ cups polenta
> 4 to 5 cups water
> Pinch of sea salt
> 2 to 3 tablespoons extra polenta, placed in a flat dish

It is not necessary to dry roast polenta first; however, it makes it taste slightly richer if you do. Make sure you warm up the frying pan first and stir the dry polenta in the hot pan.

Place water, polenta, and a pinch of sea salt in a pot. Cover. Turn the flame to medium-high; just before the water starts to bubble, turn the flame to low (it can be helpful to use a flame diffuser) and cook, covered, for about 10 to 15 minutes. Remove the polenta from the heat and put it in a dish rinsed with cold water so the polenta does not stick. Leave to cool (this may take a few hours). The deeper the dish, the longer it will take for the polenta to cool down. For this reason it's best to make it in the morning or even a day before for an evening meal.

You can refrigerate any leftover polenta and use as you desire over the course of a week. Fried polenta also makes a lovely breakfast topped with one or more of the following: honey, maple syrup, fruit purées, fresh fruit, yogurt.

BEAN AND VEGETABLE SOUP, GRILLED ZUCCHINI, AND GRATED CARROT WITH BROWN RICE VINEGAR AND BREAD WITH OLIVE OIL DIP

Start cooking the soup first; prepare the other dishes as the soup cooks.

Bean and Vegetable Soup

- 1 small carrot (2 to 3 inches), cut into squares
- 2 small cauliflower florets, broken into small pieces
- 3– to 4–inch long celery stalk, cut diagonally into slices
- 3– to 4–inch long piece of leek, shredded
- 1 small potato (or about 2–inch piece of sweet potato) cut in small squares
- 4 ounces (or ½ of a can) of navy beans (or any other type that you might have handy)
- 2 to 3 bay leaves (fresh or dried)
- Sea salt to taste
- ¼ cup of peas
- ¼ cup of fresh or canned sweet corn
- 2 small broccoli florets, broken into small pieces
- ¼ cup of small pasta shells (your choice of whole wheat, spelt, rice, or kamut)
- 1 curly kale leaf, finely shredded
- 1 to 2 tablespoons olive oil
- ½ teaspoon pesto (optional)

In a 3–quart pot place all the ingredients except for the pasta, peas, corn, broccoli, kale, olive oil, and pesto. Add 6 cups of water.

Bring to a boil and cook over a medium-high flame for 10 to 15 minutes.

Add the pasta and cook another 5 minutes. Add the peas, corn, and broccoli. Cook for a further 5 minutes. Switch off and add the kale. Season with olive oil, sea salt, and pesto (if you are using it). There is some good-quality vegan pesto on the market, which is delicious if you want to avoid cheese. Making your own pesto, in either a vegan or dairy version, is very simple, too—but it does add extra time, which can be difficult if you are in a rush.

Grilled Zucchini with Garlic, Olive Oil, and Basil

1 zucchini, around 6 to 7 inches long

½ teaspoon sea salt

1 medium clove of garlic (or more or less to taste), minced

1 tablespoon olive oil

A few basil leaves (a small handful), chopped

Cut the zucchini diagonally into pieces ⅓ inch (1 centimeter) thick. Place the slices in a flat dish and sprinkle sea salt on both sides. Leave them for 10 to 20 minutes (you will notice water sweat out of the zucchini and can do this a few hours in advance to make life easier). Heat up a skillet (or, you can cook under a grill). Place each slice in the hot skillet and cook for a few minutes on each side until brown (but not burnt).

Place in a serving dish. Mix together the olive oil, sea salt, and minced garlic and either using a brush or a small spoon, gently sprinkle the mixture over the hot zucchini. Spread the chopped basil on top.

Grated Carrot with Brown Rice Vinegar

1 small (3 to 4 inch) carrot

5 to five 6 drops brown rice vinegar

Grate the carrot very finely, so that is almost like purée. Add the brown rice vinegar and mix. Place on the serving dish next to the zucchini.

Olive Oil and Balsamic Vinegar Dip

    1 to 2 tablespoons organic cold-pressed olive oil
    1 teaspoon high-quality organic balsamic vinegar (oak-aged recommended)

Mix the olive oil and vinegar together in a small dish. Serve with a grilled sourdough baguette or some good-quality, wholesome ciabatta. Enjoy with the bean and vegetable soup. The contrast is wonderfully refreshing.

Corn, Asparagus, Tuna, Parsnip Fries, and Salad

    ½ to 1 ear of corn on the cob (depends how hungry you are)
    ¼ piece of *umeboshi*
    2 to 4 asparagus tips
    1 parsnip, around 6 inches long, cut into large matchsticks
    Olive oil for frying
    1 to 2 tablespoons of rice or chickpea flour (or you can use any other flour you
        have on hand)
    Sea salt (to taste)
    A 3– to 4–inch piece of fresh, preferably line-caught, tuna
    3 to 4 tablespoons unhulled sesame seeds (either brown or black)
    Pea-sized portion of mustard (English, French, or any other good-quality,
        sugar- and additive-free mustard that you enjoy)
    2 to 4 radishes thinly sliced
    A few fresh lettuce leaves
    Sesame or sunflower oil for seasoning (optional)
    Cress for garnishing (optional)

Pour water into a pot big enough to give the corn plenty of room. Bring to a boil over a medium to high flame and cook the corn for around 5 to 10 minutes. Take it out, let it cool for a few minutes (or until it's cool enough to handle) and then gently and lovingly rub the *umeboshi* all over it. Put it on your plate.

Use the same water to quickly blanch the asparagus for one minute (or, for a change, you could place a bamboo steamer on top of the pot and steam the asparagus for a couple of minutes). Take asparagus out and leave it to cool, or rinse it under cold water to stop it from cooking further.

Boil the parsnip matchsticks for about 5 minutes. Take them out and dry them with an unbleached paper towel or a cotton kitchen towel.

Heat up some olive oil in a skillet (you can use a bit more oil than usual, as parsnip absorbs more than most other vegetables). Combine the flour and salt, and roll each piece of parsnip in the mixture. Fry for a few minutes, turning so the parsnips gets lovely golden color on all sides.

Place them on your plate next to the corn.

Switch the flame off and swipe the skillet with a clean paper towel—make sure you have plenty of paper so you don't burn your fingers—to clean up any bits left from the parsnip. Alternatively, you could either get another skillet (if you have one) or give the one you used for the parsnip a quick wash, taking every precaution not to burn your hands.

Bring the clean skillet back onto the stove, pour in some olive oil, and heat it up. Put the sesame seeds into a flat dish and gently press each side of the tuna into them. Fry for a minute or so on each side, making sure that the middle remains raw. Take it out and put on the plate. Put mustard on top of the tuna (you can gently smear it over the surface if you'd like). Add the lettuce leaves, and place radish and asparagus on top. You can season the salad if you wish. However, both the tuna and the parsnips are quite rich, so it is nice to have something unseasoned and fresh-tasting as a contrast.

MILLET CAKES WITH PRESSED CHINESE CABBAGE SALAD AND VEGETABLE STIR-FRY

Millet Cakes

> 1 tablespoon olive oil (or toasted sesame oil, which goes especially well during cold weather)
>
> ½ cup of millet

4 to 6 cups of water (depending on the flame; millet absorbs a lot of water,
 so watch it carefully!)
¼ of a medium-sized head of cauliflower
1 tablespoon tahini
1 teaspoon *umeboshi* purée or half an *umeboshi* plum (optional)
1 to 2 tablespoons of shoyu or tamari (or sea salt to taste)
1 tablespoon pan-roasted sunflower seeds

Heat the oil briefly in a heavy pot and add the millet. Fry for 2 to 3 minutes on a
medium to high flame, stirring constantly. Add the water and place cauliflower
on top. Cover, turn the heat to low, and simmer for about 15 to 20 minutes;
check the water content from time to time and add more if necessary. The
cauliflower will almost disintegrate and millet should get soft and mushy. Add
the tahini, *umeboshi* purée (if available and desired), and shoyu and stir it all in.
Switch off the heat and let the millet stand, covered, for another 10 minutes or
so.

If the millet mixture is too soft to form into balls, make it slightly firmer by
adding a little more tahini and cooking it a little longer. Remember to keep
stirring once you add the tahini; otherwise, it sticks to the pan. When the millet
cools down, use your hands or a tablespoon to shape it into little balls. Place
them on a plate and sprinkle the pan-roasted sunflower seeds on top.

Pressed Chinese Cabbage Salad

2 to 4 Chinese cabbage leaves (depending on their size), finely chopped
Pinch of sea salt
Thinly sliced radishes, grated carrots, parsley, arugula or other leafy greens,
 and herbs, or dried sea vegetables (optional and to taste)

Place the finely chopped cabbage leaves on a plate that has a 6– to 8–inch
diameter and a bit of depth to it. Sprinkle sea salt over them. Mix gently using
your hands (please remember, this is not about squeezing the cabbage or
exercising your power) until cabbage begins to soften and feels slightly

watery (this only takes a minute or less). Put another plate on top, and then something for weight on top of that (a jar of grain, a bottle of water, anything that is stable). Leave for 10 minutes. Remove the weight, and while holding the top plate in place, drain any excess liquid. Taste the cabbage; if it's too salty, place it in a fine sieve and rinse. Drain and place on a plate to one side of the millet balls.

If you feel adventurous, you can always add thinly sliced radishes (they add lovely color), or grated carrots, parsley, fresh arugula, and any other leafy green vegetables and herbs that you like before pressing.

Another good addition would be dried sea vegetables. These come packaged in several varieties and combinations. Any combination or single sea vegetable that doesn't require cooking is fine. The one I love contains wakame, agar, and aka-tsunomata (it looks like a couple of inches of plastic strips—yet it's so delicious). All you need to do is place a teaspoon of the mixture in a tiny dish and cover it with water. In no time, it'll expand and be ready to sprinkle on your pressed Chinese cabbage for you to enjoy.

Vegetable Stir-Fry

You can use any vegetables that you like. Please consider the following to be just one example of the possibilities.

    1 to 2 tablespoons olive oil for frying
    1 each red and yellow peppers (if they're big, you can just use half of each),
        cut into strips
    4 to 6 green beans
    2– to 3–inch long carrot, cut into strips
    2– to 3–inch long piece of celery, cut into strips
    A few mushrooms (according to your appetite), sliced
    A couple of scallions, cut into thirds
    1 teaspoon shoyu or ¼ tsp sea salt for seasoning
    1 tablespoon sesame seeds

Heat up the oil in a wok or just a deep open pot. Make sure the oil isn't too hot (there should be no smoke). Add peppers and stir for a minute or two. Then add the green beans, followed by the carrots. Finally, add the celery, mushrooms, and scallions. Fry for another minute or two, stirring constantly. Season with either shoyu or sea salt. Dish out on the other side of millet and sprinkle sesame seeds all over the vegetables while they're hot.

Note: If you're trying to use as little oil as possible in your cooking, you can just brush the wok with oil to begin with and then add a few tablespoons of water along with the carrots. This keeps the vegetables from burning and helps them cook more quickly. Alternatively, you can lightly preboil any hard vegetables (carrots and green beans) and then add them after the peppers.

POTATO AND VEGETABLE SALAD WITH RICE PUDDING FOR DESSERT

Potato and Vegetable Salad

This salad makes a lovely meal. If you don't like potatoes you can leave them out and eat the salad with some cooked grain on the side. As with the stir-fry above, you can put anything you want in the salad; this is just an example.

Two handfuls of mixed fresh lettuce leaves

2 to 3 broccoli florets

2 to 3 cauliflower florets

10 green beans (fine ones go very well here), tops trimmed

Olive oil for frying and seasoning

Sea salt (to taste)

4 to 6 small new potatoes, cut into large chunks (do not peel them)

½ yellow pepper (or whole depending on size), sliced

A couple of oyster mushrooms (any other kind that you enjoy raw is fine)

2 to 3 cherry tomatoes

Balsamic vinegar (to taste)

Place the fresh lettuce leaves in a nice large bowl that you can eat out of.

Place a small pot half-filled with water over a high flame and bring it to boil. Blanch the broccoli, cauliflower, and green beans (only one kind at a time) for a minute or less; leave them on a plate to cool down. If you're in a hurry, rinse them with cold water.

Use the same water to boil the potatoes. This should take 5 minutes or so. Take them out and dry them with a kitchen towel.

Heat up the olive oil in a skillet and fry the potatoes for a few minutes on each side until they get a lovely golden color. Just before they're finished, sprinkle them with sea salt. Keep them in the skillet while you arrange the rest of the salad.

Place all the cooked vegetables and the peppers, mushrooms, and tomatoes around the bowl adding the potatoes last. They are nice warm; however, if they're too hot they'll wilt the lettuce leaves. Season the salad with olive oil and balsamic vinegar.

Use your imagination and desire when it comes to choosing what to put in the salad. Some suggestions: snap peas, snow peas, corn, asparagus, cabbage, and radishes.

Rice Pudding

Makes enough for several people and will last several days refrigerated.

> 3½ ounces almonds (or hazelnuts or walnuts)
> 7 ounces precooked sweet brown rice (or short-grain brown rice)
> 2 pints vanilla (or plain) rice milk
> 3½ ounces raisins
> ½ small orange (zest and juice)
> 3 tablespoons honey (or maple syrup)
> A few drops of vanilla extract
> A sprinkle of cinnamon

Dry roast the nuts by placing them in a dry skillet over low heat and stirring until lightly toasted on both sides. This should take 2 to 4 minutes. Roughly chop the nuts and put them aside, keeping a few whole for decoration.

Mix the precooked rice and rice milk together in a medium saucepan. Bring to a boil, reduce the heat to medium-low, and simmer for 10 to 20 minutes. Add the raisins. Grate the orange zest, squeeze the juice, and add them to the saucepan. Simmer for a few more minutes. Add the honey and vanilla extract and turn off the heat. Serve the pudding warm in individual bowls with a sprinkle of cinnamon and a few whole nuts.

CHAPTER FORTY-SEVEN

Dinners

MISO SOUP, BROWN BASMATI RICE, AND THAI COCONUT STEW WITH PRESSED CUCUMBER, DAIKON, AND BEETS

Miso Soup

> 3 cups of water
>
> 1 small onion, chopped
>
> 1 medium carrot, cut into sticks
>
> 2–inch piece of dried wakame
>
> 1 teaspoon miso (any kind is fine, and it's good to eat a variety)
>
> A few drops of olive oil
>
> A handful of watercress, finely chopped
>
> ¼ sheet of nori, cut into fine strips

Bring the water to a boil. Add the onions and simmer for 2 to 3 minutes. Add the carrots and simmer for another 2 minutes. Switch off the heat. Break the wakame into small pieces and add it to the soup. Take another, smaller pot and ladle one soup portion into it. Leave the rest to cool and then refrigerate. (Every day, you can dish out enough for one serving and continue the recipe from this point. This way your miso soup will always be fresh.)

In a cup or a small bowl, mix 1 teaspoon of miso and couple of tablespoons of cold water. Make sure all the bits are broken into a smooth paste.

Add a small handful of watercress to the small pot of soup. Serve the soup into a bowl. Add the diluted miso to bowl and mix. Add a few drops of olive oil. Top with nori and serve.

Note: There are many options you can add to miso soup. If you like, and particularly during colder days, you can add some grated garlic and ginger to the soup at the same time as the watercress. It tastes richer and it is beautifully warming. Chunks of tofu go well in this soup, too. For nonvegetarians, I highly recommend you add mussels, clams, or pieces of fresh white fish several times a week.

A word of advice: Make sure that you don't overheat the miso. Miso is rich in enzymes, and it is thought that high temperatures destroy some of them. Also, watch for the amount of miso you add. Remember that it is quite salty, so too much miso can have an adverse effect.

This particular miso soup is the traditional kind, but any soup can be made into miso soup by adding miso, which is fermented soybean paste. Miso contains live cultures and it is brilliant for digestion and recommended for anyone recovering from an illness.

Brown Basmati Rice

> 1 cup brown basmati rice
> water

First, rinse the rice in 2 or 3 changes of water. Put the rice in a pot and add water to just cover it. Leave it to soak for at least 5 hours. You can do this in the morning if you are planning on having it for lunch or dinner, or you can even do it the night before.

When you're ready for dinner, bring the rice to a boil, reduce the flame to medium-low, and simmer, covered, for 15 to 20 minutes. Please check the water level periodically; if your flame is too high and water is evaporating rapidly, you might need to add a little bit of water during the course of cooking. It's always better to start with less water and keep adding than the opposite. If you start with more water, your rice is likely to get overcooked and often ends up being soggy.

If you like, you can add a pinch of salt to it during the cooking. In my family, if we are eating it with a bean stew that is seasoned, we prefer to have our rice unseasoned.

A good thing about rice is that you can cook enough for a few servings and then vary how you use the rest: in soups, fried, stews, with a vegetable stir-fry, or baked. This way you save time on cooking, which means you can have a healthy, tasty meal in a very short time.

Michael and Georgina's Thai Coconut Stew

1 to 2 tablespoons organic cold-pressed extra virgin olive oil

2 to 3 cloves of garlic, minced

1 small onion, diced

1 small red pepper, diced (optional)

1 small carrot (about 4 inches) cut into squares

1 can organic chickpeas (or any other kind that you like), rinsed

1 small package of deep-fried tofu (approximately 8 ounces),
   cut into small cubes

½ jar of good organic Thai green curry sauce (or 1 tablespoon
   Thai green curry paste mixed with water)

½ teaspoon kudzu, arrowroot, or cornstarch for thickening, mixed into
   a small amount of warm water

Sea salt

1 cup canned organic coconut milk (nonorganic versions on the market often
   have lots of junk in them, so please read the label carefully)

Large bunch of cilantro, finely chopped

When Michael, our youngest son (who was 11 at the time), stayed with Simon's niece (who is a year his senior) and then got back home, he volunteered to prepare dinner for us using the recipe that the two of them had come up with. This is their recipe. The curry that we use is so beautifully fragrant and not too spicy, full of lime and lemongrass.

Heat up the olive oil in a heavy pot. Do not let it smoke. Add the garlic and onions and sauté for a few minutes. Add the pepper, keep stirring, and then add carrots after a few minutes. Sauté further, then add the chickpeas and tofu. Keep sautéing it all for 5 to 10 minutes, and then add the curry sauce.

If necessary, you can add a touch of water to stop ingredients from sticking to the pan.

Add your thickener, season with sea salt, add coconut milk, and simmer to heat everything through. Just before serving, switch off the heat and throw in a very generous amount of cilantro (go over the top—it cannot spoil this dish).

Serve on organic brown basmati rice—delicious. It must be the richness of coconut milk that attracts all the flavor. The whole dish is a 10–minute job. It tastes as good, if not better, the next day or even few days later. I always try to make enough so that there are leftovers, but not with our hungry tribe. If you're making enough for a few servings, do not pour in all the coconut milk as instructed above. Instead, take enough for one serving, put it in another pot, and add a smaller amount of coconut milk. Refrigerate the rest (only after it has completely cooled down) and add coconut milk toward the end each time you heat some up. This stops it from getting spoiled too soon.

Pressed Cucumber, Daikon, and Beets

A 5– to 6–inch cucumber, cut in half and then thinly sliced
2 inches of daikon (or 6 to 8 radishes), thinly sliced into half moons
¼ teaspoon sea salt
1 tablespoon pickled, raw, or cooked grated beets

Place the cucumber and daikon in a deep plate, sprinkle with salt, and work gently with your hands for a minute. Put another flat plate on top and place a weight (about 2 pounds) on top (use a bottle or a jar or something similar). Let stand for 10 to 15 minutes. Take the weight off, but keep the plate. Hold the plates firmly together and tip them over a sink to get rid of excess water. Place the cucumber and daikon in a serving bowl and add the beets. This salad is very refreshing and delicious as it is, but if you like you can season it with a dressing before serving. We also like it with a few pan-roasted sunflower seeds or crushed pan-roasted sesame seeds (black or brown).

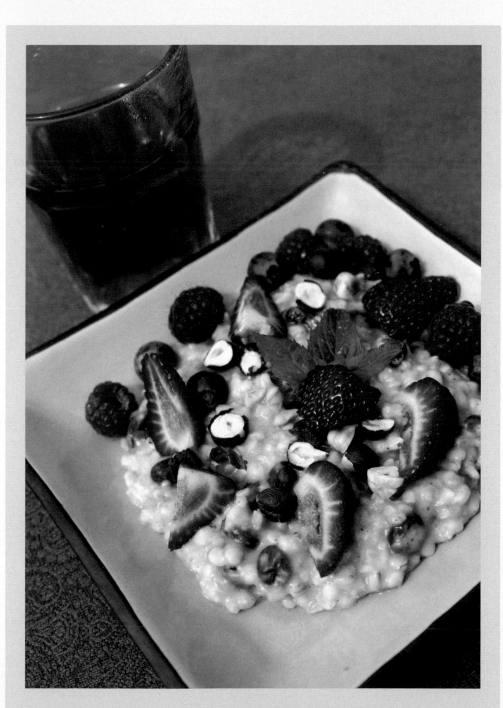

Whole oat porridge, berries and nuts, and hot kukicha.
See page 295 for recipes.

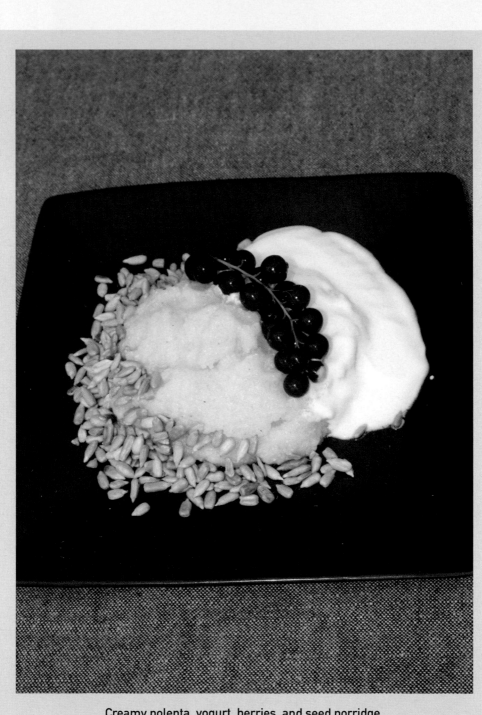

Creamy polenta, yogurt, berries, and seed porridge.
See page 297 for recipes.

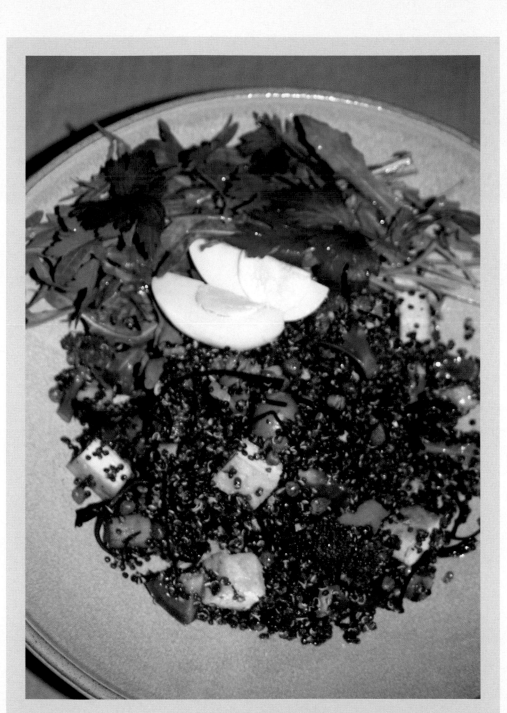

Red quinoa, tofu, and vegetable salad with fresh green herbs and egg.
See pages 298–299 for recipes.

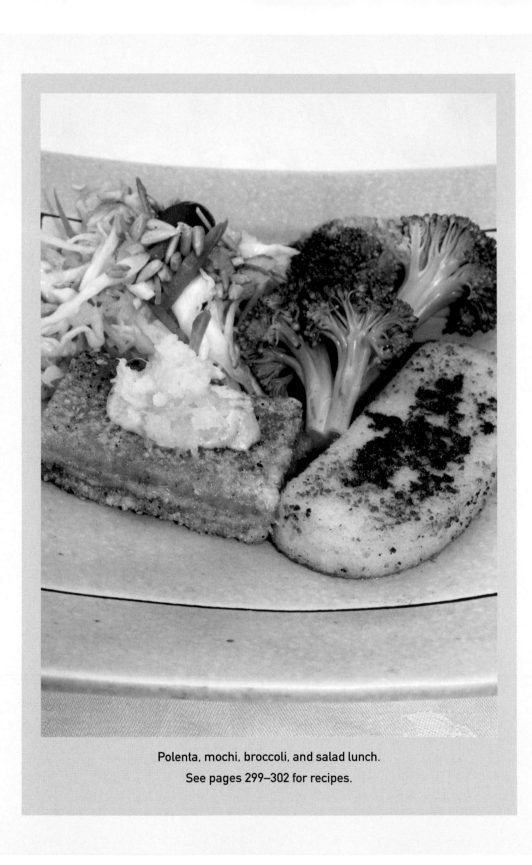

Polenta, mochi, broccoli, and salad lunch.
See pages 299–302 for recipes.

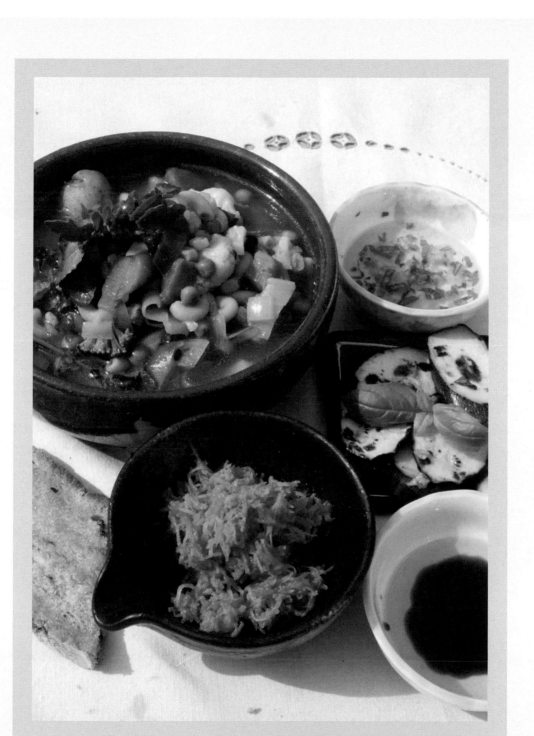

Bean and vegetable soup, grilled zucchini, and grated carrot with brown rice vinegar and bread with olive oil dip. See pages 302–304 for recipes.

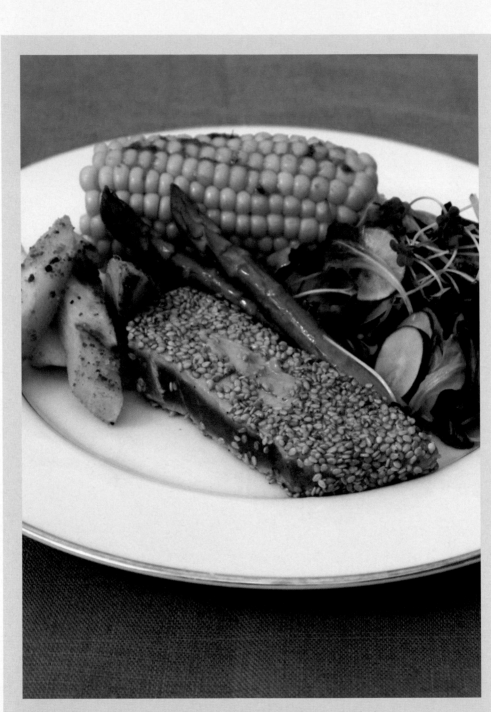

Corn, asparagus, tuna, parsnip fries, and salad.
See pages 304–305 for recipes.

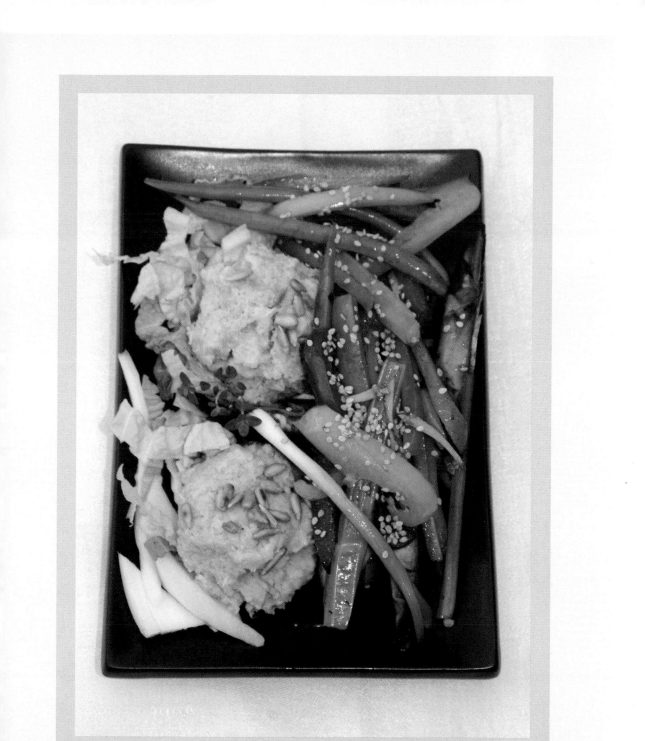

Millet cakes with pressed Chinese cabbage salad and vegetable stir-fry.
See pages 305–308 for recipes.

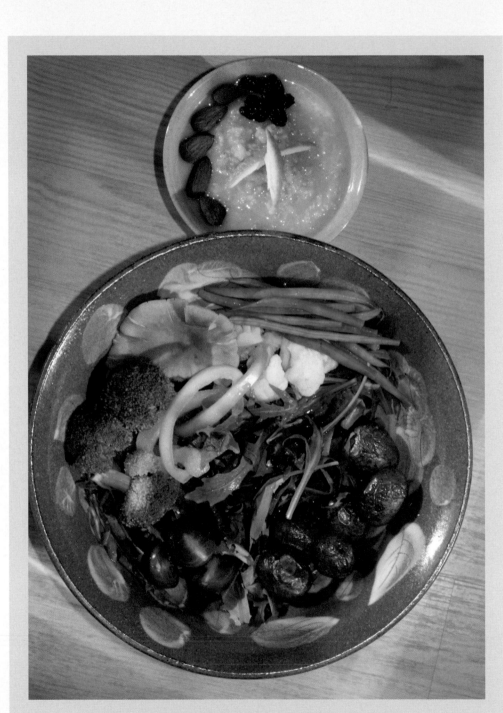

Potato and vegetable salad with rice pudding for dessert.
See pages 308–310 for recipes.

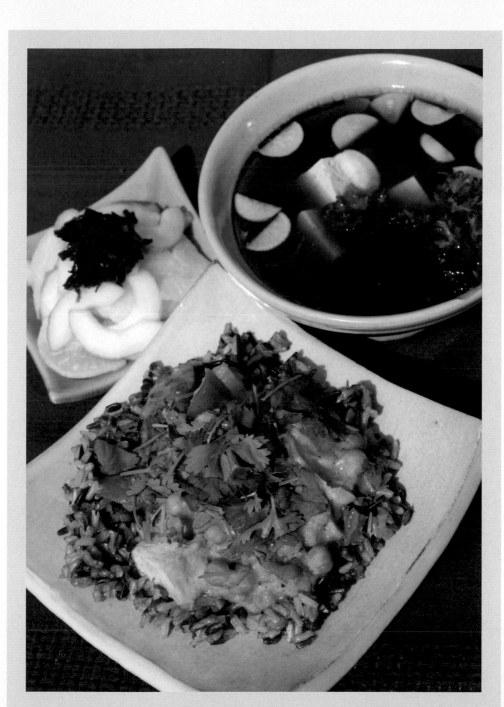

Miso soup, brown basmati rice, and Thai coconut stew with pressed cucumber, daikon, and beets. See pages 311–314 for recipes.

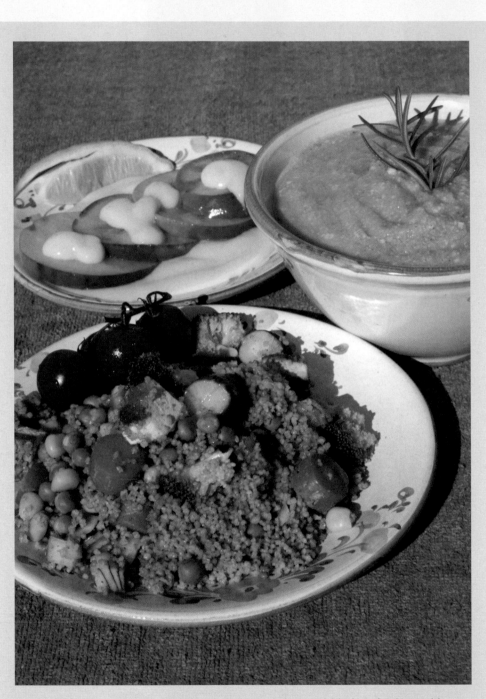

Cauliflower and lentil dahl soup, couscous salad, and fried apple rings with vanilla pudding for dessert. See pages 315–316 for recipes.

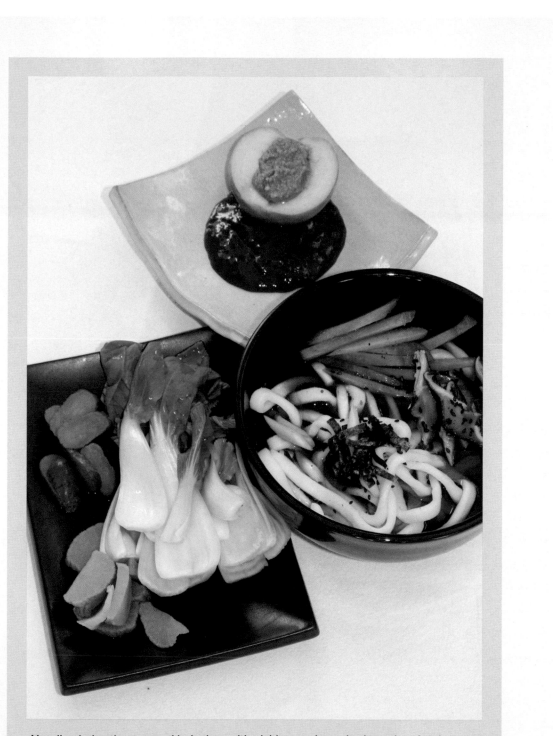

Noodles in broth, steamed bok choy with pickles, and poached peaches for dessert.
See pages 317–319 for recipes.

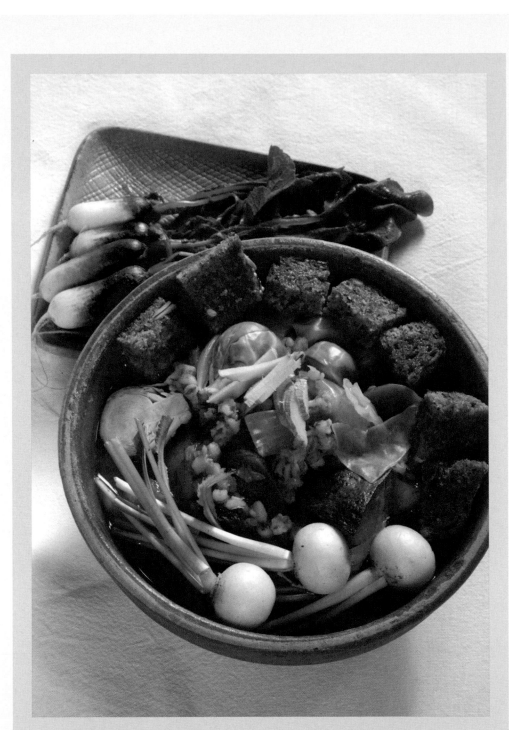

Barley and vegetable stew with fried bread and blanched radishes.
See pages 320–321 for recipes.

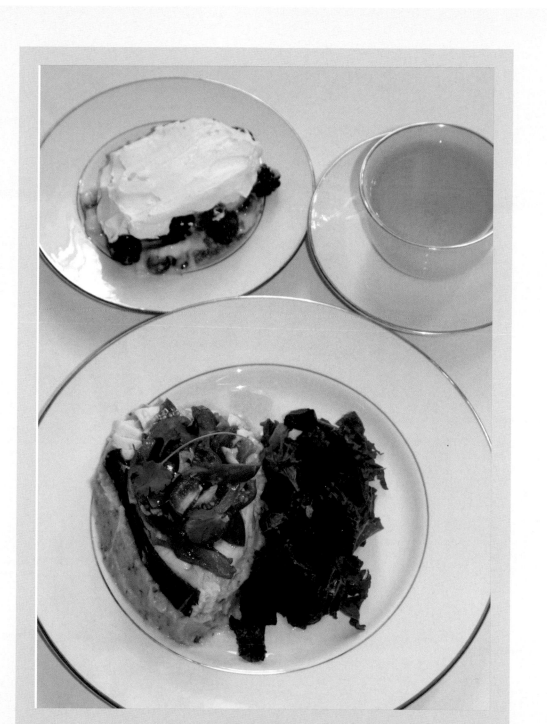

Steamed fish on a bed of butter beans, kale and beets,and
Banoffee pie for dessert. See pages 321–324 for recipes.

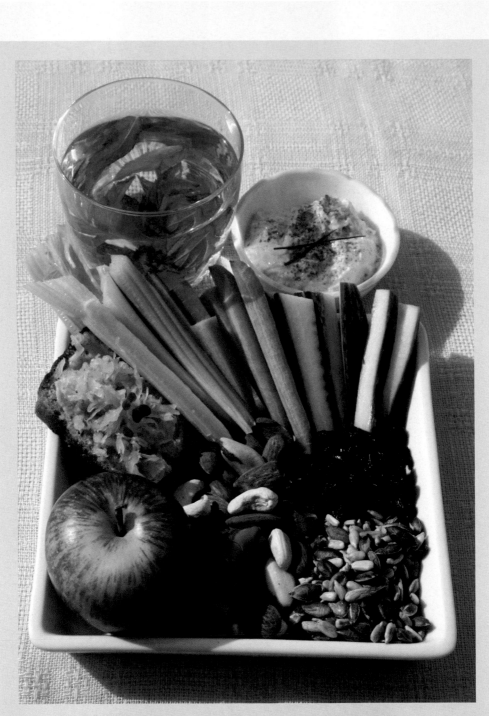

A range of healthy macrobiotic snacks and fresh mint tea.
See pages 325–326 for recipes.

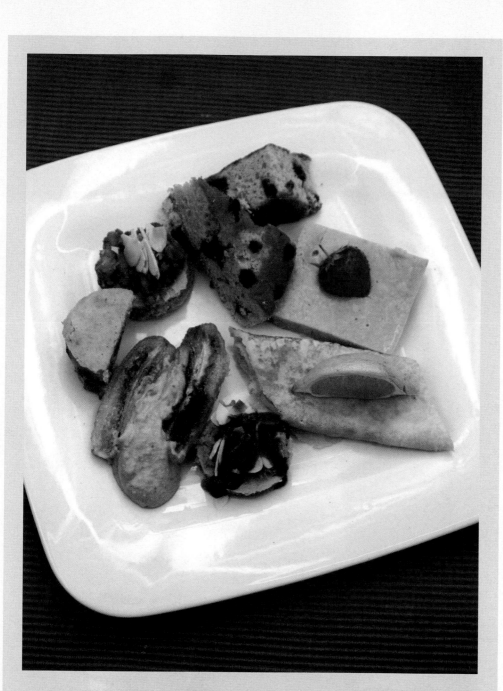

Cakes and other desserts: pancakes, orange amasake pudding, fried banana with cashew and berry cream, cherry cake, and parachutes with orange-nut topping. See pages 327–330 for recipes.

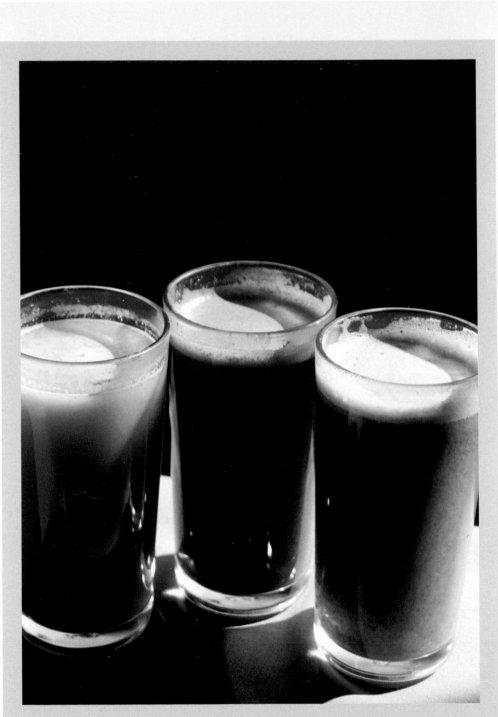

Fresh red, golden, and green vegetable and fruit juices.
See pages 331–332 for recipes.

CAULIFLOWER AND LENTIL DAHL SOUP, COUSCOUS SALAD, AND FRIED APPLE RINGS WITH VANILLA PUDDING FOR DESSERT

Cauliflower and Lentil Dahl Soup

1 cup of red lentils

4 ounces of tofu

1 very small cauliflower

1 tablespoon organic korma or tikka masala paste

1 tablespoon olive oil plus more for frying garlic (optional)

A few garlic cloves, sliced (optional)

Sea salt to taste

Wash the lentils and place them in a saucepan together with the tofu, cauliflower, and korma. Cover with twice as much water as the volume of your other ingredients and bring it to a boil. Simmer until lentils are cooked. Keep checking that there is enough water, but not too much. Remove from heat, blend, and season with sea salt and olive oil. If the soup is too thick, add more water to get the consistency you like. You can also fry a few sliced garlic cloves in little olive oil and add to the soup at the end.

Couscous Salad

9 ounces tofu, cut into ½-inch squares

5 tablespoons shoyu

1 tablespoon brown rice vinegar

1½ cup couscous (you could make this with 1 cup quinoa instead; see alternate instructions below)

3 cups water

1 small onion, diced

1 small carrot (4–5 inches), diced

A 4- to 5-inch celery stalk, diced

3 ounces peas

3 ounces sweet corn

A few strands of chive for garnish

Marinate the tofu for 10 minutes in the brown rice vinegar and 2 tablespoons of the shoyu, stirring occasionally.

Bring the water to a boil in a saucepan. Add a pinch of sea salt. Add the couscous and switch off the heat. Cover and let stand; the couscous will cook without external heat in about 20 minutes. (If you're using quinoa, bring 2 cups of water to a boil and add the grain; cover, simmer, and cook for approximately 15 minutes.) Once the couscous or quinoa is cooked, let it cool and fluff it up with a fork before mixing with the other ingredients.

Meanwhile, heat the oil in a large, heavy pan and add the marinated tofu. Add the onion and the sea salt (dip the tips of chopsticks in salt, and then use them to stir the onion). Pan-fry for a few minutes, stirring constantly. Add the carrots and celery and stir until mixed well with the rest. Cook for a few more minutes then add the peas and sweet corn. Cook for another 3 to 4 minutes and turn the heat off. Mix the couscous in. Season with the rest of the shoyu. Garnish with few chive strands.

Fried Apple Rings with Vanilla Pudding

1 apple, cored and sliced into ¼-inch rings

Olive oil for frying

A sprinkle of cinnamon (optional)

Vanilla pudding, store-bought or packaged (follow package instructions to prepare; if you're vegan you can make it with a grain or nut milk instead of any dairy milk that's called for)

Heat up a little bit of olive oil in a frying pan; gently fry the apple rings for a few minutes on each side. Cover a small plate with some vanilla pudding. Put the hot fried apple rings on top. Sprinkle with cinnamon if desired.

NOODLES IN BROTH, STEAMED BOK CHOY WITH PICKLES, AND POACHED PEACHES FOR DESSERT

Noodles in Broth

8 ounces rice, buckwheat or wheat noodles (or more or less, depending on
   how hungry you are)

4 cups water

1 3–inch strip of kombu

4 small dried shiitake mushrooms

A pinch of sea salt

1 cup bonito flakes (optional—see note below)

1 small onion, sliced into half-moons

1 medium carrot, cut into matchsticks

4 to 5 tablespoons shoyu or tamari

1 small scallion, chopped fine

1 tablespoon toasted sesame seeds

½ sheet nori, cut into strips

Shichimi (Japanese seven spice powder) to taste (optional)

Cook the noodles according to the package instructions. When they're done, rinse them under cold water.

Meanwhile, or even before, start making a broth. Place 4 cups of water into a large saucepan; bring to a boil, and add the kombu, mushrooms, and sea salt. Place bonito flakes in a sieve that fits into the pot, put inside and cover.

Simmer for 15 minutes. Take out and discard the bonito flakes. Take out the kombu and chop it. Take out the mushrooms, discard the stems, and slice the caps. Put the mushrooms and chopped kombu back in the pan. Add the onion and cook for 5 minutes. Add the carrot and cook for another 2 minutes. Turn off the heat, then season the broth with shoyu. (If you're in a hurry you can skip the onions and the carrots; however, it is worth the effort. The vegetables in this dish absorb the strong tastes and smells from the bonito, shiitakes, and shoyu, and they taste delicious.)

When just ready to serve, dip the noodles into hot water to reheat them, then drain and place in a large bowl. Pour the broth and contents of the broth over the noodles. Sprinkle some scallions on top and a generous spoonful of sesame seeds. Garnish with nori strips and *shichimi.*

You can add large cubes of tofu at the end if you like. For greater richness you can fry the tofu first. Fresh sea food like cockles and mussels are a great addition too.

Note: Dried bonito flakes, known as *katsuo-bushi* or *katsuobushi* in Japan, are flakes of dried, fermented, and smoked skipjack tuna. They look similar to very fine wood shavings. Bonito flakes are often used to make dashi, a broth that is the basis for miso soup. They can also be used as filling for rice balls. If you are vegan, vegetarian, or cannot get bonito flakes, leave them out of this recipe.

Steamed Bok Choy with Pickles

Handful of bok choy
1–inch piece of pickled daikon (*takuan*) or any other pickle, finely sliced
1 or 2 small gherkins, roughly chopped

Place a pot that holds 1 pint of water and fits with a bamboo steamer (if you haven't got one you can use a metal steamer, just make sure to use less water so that it is not touching the vegetables, otherwise they get too soggy) on the burner. Turn the flame on high and wait for the water to start boiling. Turn the flame down to medium and place the bamboo steamer, with the bok choy inside, carefully on top of the pot. If you are using a metal steamer that goes inside a pot, I suggest you use very long chopsticks or long tongs to place the bok choy inside to avoid getting burned by the steam.

Steam bok choy for 1 minute. Bok choy leaves are soft and succulent, and they cook very quickly; the stalks will remain crunchy. The combination is delicious.

Take it out and place on a serving plate. You can sprinkle some oil on top, or leave as is. Next to it, place the cut-up pickles. These can be bought in good health food stores. Make sure you read the ingredients, though, to avoid sugar and/or any other artificial flavors, colors, etc.

Poached Peaches

Makes two servings.

    2 peaches, cut in half

    ½ cup each cranberry and apple juice

    Pinch of sea salt

    1 tablespoon honey or maple syrup

    1¼ to 1½ ounces roasted ground almonds

    1 teaspoon kudzu or arrowroot

    1 teaspoon grated lemon zest

Place peaches face-up in a pan and pour the juices on top. Bring to a boil. Reduce flame to medium. Add a pinch of sea salt. Cook for 2 to 3 minutes (they should remain firm). Cooking time largely depends on the kind of peaches and how ripe they are; soft ones might take only a minute or so, whereas the hard ones will take a little longer. In either case, the objective is to have them firm rather than too soft. Take the peaches out and place them on a plate to cool down. Reserve the juice.

Heat the honey or syrup and add the almonds. Stir until the mixture thickens. Put one teaspoon into the hollow of each peach.

Briefly simmer the reserved cranberry and apple juice with kudzu to thicken it; add the lemon zest. Divide the thickened juice into two small bowls. Place two peach halves into each bowl and enjoy. You can keep the leftover serving out of the refrigerator until the next day unless the room is very hot; if it's hot or if you might not eat it for two days, refrigerate it and take it out couple of hours before serving.

BARLEY AND VEGETABLE STEW WITH FRIED BREAD AND BLANCHED RADISHES

Barley Stew

> 7 ounces barley, washed and presoaked for a few hours
>
> A 2–inch piece of leek, diced (or use a small onion if leeks are not available)
>
> 1 small carrot, diced
>
> 6 to 8 ounces kabocha pumpkin when in season (otherwise, use any other pumpkin)
>
> ½ celery stalk, diced
>
> A couple of baby turnips (or a few chunks of ordinary turnip)
>
> 2 to 3 brussels sprouts
>
> Sea salt or miso
>
> 1 slice of sourdough, natural-rise rice bread (or any other whole-grain bread)
>
> Olive oil for frying the bread
>
> 1 large garlic clove, cut in half
>
> Parsley for garnish

Cook barley in twice its volume of water for 20 minutes to half an hour. Every now and again, check to make sure that there is enough water. You can always do this a day in advance.

Lay the ingredients in a heavy cast iron pot in the following order: leek, carrot, pumpkin, celery, and precooked barley. Cover with water, and cook for 15 minutes or so, adding water from time to time only if necessary. Add the turnips and brussels sprouts, and cook 10 minutes more. Season with sea salt or miso. Always put in a small amount of seasoning, taste the dish, and then add more if necessary. Simmer the stew for a couple more minutes, switch off the heat, and cover.

Pour olive oil into a skillet (preferably cast iron) to just cover the surface. Over a medium to high flame, fry the bread for a couple of minutes on each side.

Take the bread out of the skillet and, while the bread is very hot, rub the cut garlic clove on both sides. (It may be easiest to do this with the garlic on the end of a fork.) Put it in a bowl type dish, pour the stew on top and decorate with a few parsley leaves. If you prefer your bread to be crunchier, you can put it on top of the stew.

The stew should be creamy and moist but not watery. This is a good cold-weather dish. Its creamy quality is very relaxing. Stews are extremely practical, because you can make enough for a few servings and they are cheap to make yet substantial. Keep adding different vegetables, whatever tickles your fancy. At the end of cooking, experiment with adding scallions, Chinese cabbage, bok choy, savoy cabbage, carrot tops, or anything else that sounds appealing to you.

Blanched Radishes

4 to 5 radishes (or as many as you can eat with this stew) with their greens on

Place a small pot on the stove and fill it with about an inch of water.

Bring to a boil, add the radishes and cover; cook for a minute or less. Switch off the heat, scoop out the radishes, and place them on a serving dish. If you're eating them with the stew, there's no need to add any seasoning since the stew is rich. However, if you're having them on their own or with another dish that's not so rich, you can add few drops of any oil that you like and a few drops of fresh-squeezed lemon or orange juice.

STEAMED FISH ON A BED OF BUTTER BEANS, KALE AND BEETS, AND BANOFFEE PIE FOR DESSERT

Butter Bean Mash

7 ounces canned butter beans (or precooked if you have any)
2 tablespoons olive oil
⅛ cup of water
Handful of fresh basil leaves
Pinch of sea salt

Place the beans and water in a small pot and bring to a boil. Switch off heat and pour into a blender. Blend to smooth consistency. Add sea salt, basil, and olive oil and gently blend for 10 seconds. Taste and if necessary add more salt, olive oil, or water, depending how creamy or thick you like it.

Steamed Fish

1 halibut steak (or any other white fish)

1 small onion, sliced

2 bay leaves

4 to 5 cherry tomatoes, halved or quartered

1 clove of garlic, crushed

1 to 2 tablespoons olive oil

¼ teaspoon sea salt

1 small red, yellow, or green pepper, roasted and sliced (see note)

A handful of fresh cilantro, chopped

Fill a small pot halfway with water and place it on the stove. Add the onion and bay leaves. Bring to a boil and simmer for 5 minutes; the bay and onions will begin to give off a lovely smell. Drop the fish in the water and boil for a few minutes. If the fish is very fresh, it should only take a minute or two. If you leave it in too long, it will begin to disintegrate.

While that's simmering, in another little pot place tomatoes, garlic, olive oil, sea salt, and peppers. Turn the heat on and warm up, but do not boil. Turn the heat off and add the cilantro, leaving a little aside for a garnish. Place the pureed beans on the plate roughly in the shape of the fish, place the fish on the beans, put the vegetables on top, and sprinkle with the remaining cilantro. Serve immediately.

Note: To roast a pepper, you can use the oven, the grill, or the stovetop (with a flame diffuser). Heat the whole pepper until its skin is charred, making sure to apply heat to all sides. Put it in a dish and wrap a kitchen towel around it so that it sweats (this makes it easier to peel). When the pepper is cool enough to handle, peel it and discard the stem and seeds; you can also rinse it in cold water to make sure there are no seeds or black bits left. This is best done in advance (even a couple of days earlier than you will be using it is fine).

Boiled Kale and Beets

2 to 3 large leaves of green curly kale, stems removed and leaves chopped

1 to 2 small beets, precooked (boiled until soft) and cubed

Bring some water to a boil in a small pot. Add the kale and cook for a minute or so. The kale's color should intensify, but it should not get soggy. Drain the kale and put the beet on top. You can dress this dish, but because the fish has olive oil and garlic and tastes rich, I prefer to leave the vegetables as they are.

Banoffee Pie

6 sugar-free cookies

1 tablespoon butter

1 cup vanilla pudding, store-bought or packaged (follow package instructions to prepare)

4 to 6 cups or 2 pounds of mixed berries (for example, raspberries, blueberries, and gooseberries)

1 large banana, sliced

1 small package of whipping cream (optional, for dairy lovers!)

Place a clean kitchen towel on a large chopping board or similar flat surface. Place the cookies on top and fold the towel in half; gently press the cookies with a rolling pin through the towel until they are broken up into powder, with some larger bits remaining.

Melt the butter in a small saucepan. Add the cookie crumbs and mix with a fork until fully moistened. Place the mixture in a flat dish a couple of inches deep. With your hands, press the crumb and butter mixture into a thin layer at the bottom of the dish; refrigerate for half an hour or until it is nice and firm.

Take it out, spread the vanilla pudding on top, and refrigerate for another 10 minutes; then, place all the fruits on top.

If you are using cream, put it on top; if not, enjoy as it is.

CHAPTER FORTY-EIGHT

Snacks

Fresh Mint Tea

> 6 to 10 fresh mint leaves
> Lemon (optional)
> Honey (optional)

Place mint leaves in a cup and pour hot water over them. Squeeze in lemon for added zest and to make the tea even more alkaline-forming. Add honey if you want a more soothing tea.

Bread Snack

> Sourdough rye bread or any whole-grain bread
> Tahini (or any nut butter)
> Sauerkraut

Steam or toast the bread, and spread tahini (or any nut butter) on it; top with sauerkraut. For a sweeter version, use sugar-free jam or honey instead of sauerkraut.

Crudités and Hummus

> Cucumber, celery, and carrots, sliced into 2–inch strips
> Hummus, premade
> Turmeric
> Chive, scallion, sage, or any other herbs of your choice, chopped (optional)

Place hummus in a dish and sprinkle on turmeric to taste. Add herbs, if using. Dip vegetables into the hummus and eat. This is a great snack to keep your blood sugar stable.

Trail Mix

Almonds, hazelnuts, peanuts, cashews, Brazil nuts, walnuts, and/or pecans
Sunflower and/or pumpkin seeds
Dried fruit, such as raisins

Mix the nuts and seeds of your choice with dried fruit to make a satisfying snack. If you want a crunchier texture and a richer taste, you can roast the seeds and any of the nuts (except cashews and Brazil nuts). Heat up a large pan or skillet and place the nuts or seeds in until they begin to change color. Pumpkin seeds will expand and pop.

Fresh Fruit

Any fresh fruit

Most fresh fruit is best eaten with the skin on. Eating some raw foods will complement the cooked part of your diet. Fruits are generally alkaline-forming, and are better than many snacks in terms of maintaining stable blood sugar levels. They are whole and full of living energy.

CHAPTER FORTY-NINE

Cakes and Other Desserts

Pancakes

2 cups flour (any you like)

Pinch of sea salt

1 egg, beaten

2¼ cups still or sparkling mineral water

1 tablespoon olive oil

Mix flour and sea salt in a medium mixing bowl. Make a depression in the middle and add the egg and a small amount of the water. Begin stirring, and stir constantly as you continue to add water a little at a time. When you have added about 1¼ cups of water, you should have a wet but firm dough. At this point, pound it with wooden spoon for a few minutes and make sure there are no lumps. Then, thin it down with the remaining water. Let the batter rest in the refrigerator for about 15 minutes. Add olive oil, mix well. Meanwhile, heat a tablespoon of oil in a cast-iron skillet and, when the oil is hot but not smoking, take a ladle full of batter, spread it around the skillet, and fry for 2 to 4 minutes. Turn the pancake over and fry it for another 2 to 4 minutes on the second side.

Fill pancakes with sugar-free jam or honey and lemon juice.

Orange Amasake Pudding

2 cups sugar-free exotic juice (mango, papaya, and/or similar;
a mixture works well)

2 cups amasake

1 cup water

4 tablespoon agar agar

1 to 2 tablespoons honey or maple syrup

1 teaspoon vanilla extract

½ cup ground dry-roasted almonds

1 orange

Berries for garnish

Place the juice, amasake, water, and agar agar in a pot. Bring to a boil on a medium to low flame and simmer for 10 minutes or until the agar is dissolved. Add the honey or maple syrup and vanilla and mix gently. Turn off the heat and pour the mixture into a dish. Add the almonds, stirring well, and leave to set. Grate the zest of the orange; then squeeze the juice into a dish. (If you freeze the orange for 10 to 15 minutes first, it is much easier to grate it.) When the pudding is half set (test it by gently putting your finger on top of mixture and feeling for a light skin), mix in the orange zest and juice. Leave it to fully set. This may take an hour or more. Place in individual dishes, garnish with a berry, and serve.

Fried Banana with Cashew and Berry Cream

¼ cup cashews

¼ to ½ cup sugar-free apple juice

2 tablespoons maple syrup

¼ cup blueberries (or raspberries or strawberries, or a mixture)

1 banana, cut in half

1 teaspoon olive oil for frying

Put the cashews into a small saucepan with about a cup of water. Bring to a boil and simmer for 10 minutes or so. Add more water if necessary. Drain the cashews and put them in a blender. Add a small amount of apple juice and the maple syrup, and blend. Keeping adding more juice as required to get a smooth consistency. Finally, add the berries and blend briefly.

Heat up the oil in a frying pan, and fry the banana halves for 2 to 3 minutes on each side. Place in a long dish and pour the cashew and berry cream over them.

Cherry Cake

1 large organic free-range egg

½ cup maple syrup

1 cup coconut oil

1 cup rice milk

2 tablespoons baking powder

4 cups flour (any kind; gluten-free flour makes this pie lighter)

1 cup sweet or sour pitted cherries

Whisk the egg and maple syrup together for a minute or so. Add the rest of the ingredients except for cherries and mix well.

Preheat oven to 350°. Oil a baking dish and add in half the batter. Bake for 5 to 10 minutes, until cake starts to become firm. Take out of oven and place cherries on top of the cake; then pour the other half of the batter over them. Bake for another 15 to 20 minutes.

If you are unsure whether it's ready, stick a toothpick into the top layer of cake. If it emerges without batter sticking to it, the cake is ready.

PARACHUTES WITH ORANGE-NUT TOPPING

Parachutes

2 organic free-range eggs

½ cup maple syrup

1 cup coconut oil

1 cup rice milk

1 tablespoon baking powder

2 cups flour

Mix the eggs and maple syrup for a few minutes. Add coconut oil and rice milk and mix for another minute. Add baking powder and flour and mix till there are no lumps.

Preheat oven to 350°. Oil a 13x9x2–inch baking dish, pour the mixture in, and bake for 15 to 20 minutes. When it cools down, take the pastry out of the dish and place it on a chopping board. Get a small glass (about 1½ inches in diameter) and, holding it upside-down, use it to cut the pastry into circles. Place the circles of pastry on a serving dish. Keep the remaining pastry for the topping.

Orange-Nut Topping

> ½ cup apple juice
>
> ¼ cup maple syrup
>
> ¼ cup walnuts, hazelnuts, and/or almonds, roughly chopped
>
> Juice of ½ freshly squeezed orange
>
> ½ tablespoon grated orange zest
>
> Reserved pastry from the Parachutes recipe
>
> ½ cup slivered almond for decoration

Mix together the apple juice, maple syrup, chopped nuts, orange juice, and orange zest. Using your hands, crumble up the leftovers from the pastry and combine it with the juice-nut mixture. Spoon the topping onto the Parachutes. Decorate with slivered almonds.

CHAPTER FIFTY
Fresh Vegetable and Fruit Juices

The instructions for all of the following juices are the same: Put the vegetables and fruits through your juicer and drink right away. I don't wash or peel vegetables or fruits that are organic and look clean. You can mix any juice with hot water to give yourself a more relaxing feeling. These juices are highly alkaline-forming and full of fresh nutrients.

Fresh Red Juice

> 2 apples
> 2 carrots
> 1 small beet
> 1 small pear

Fresh Golden Juice

> 1 apple
> 3 carrots
> 1 large orange
> ¼ small lemon
> ¼ inch piece of fresh ginger root

Fresh Green Juice

> 2 sweet green apples
> 1 celery stalk
> Handful of mint
> 1 small lime or lemon

Fresh Intuitive Juice

12 breaths with focus

1 meditation

As much living in the moment as you like

Feel what combination of vegetables and fruits will make your ideal juice.

CONTRIBUTORS' WEB SITES
AND E-MAIL ADDRESSES

Herman Aihara
  www.vega.macrobiotic.net/index.htm

Leslie Ashburn
  leslie@macrobiotichawaii.com
  www.macrobiotichawaii.com

Serge Benhayon
  serge@universalmedicine.com.au
  http://universalmedicine.com.au/

David Briscoe
  david@macroamerica.com
  www.macroamerica.com/index.php

Dragana Brown
  dragana@chienergy.co.uk
  www.lusciousorganic.co.uk/

Melanie Brown Waxman
  info@celebrate4health.com
  www.celebrate4health.com/

Simon Brown
  simon@chienergy.co.uk
  www.chienergy.co.uk/

Bob Carr
  RNCJR@apk.net
  http://junior.apk.net/~rncjr

Carl Ferré
gomf@earthlink.net
www.gomf.macrobiotic.net/

Greg Johnson
gregjohnson@concordinstitute.com
www.concordinstitute.com/

Michio Kushi
www.michiokushi.org/
www.kushiinstitute.org/

Norio Kushi
organicwheels@gmail.com
www.demystifyenlightenment.org/

Phiya Kushi
phiyak@gmail.com
www.phiya.com/

Anna Mackenzie
anna@annamackenzie.co.uk
www.macrobiotics.org.uk/

Meredith McCarty
meredith@healingcuisine.com
www.healingcuisine.com/

Jan Mosbacher
http://hubpages.com/profile/Jan+Mosbacher

Andy Nicola
andy@andynicolaastrology.com
www.andynicolaastrology.com/

Jadranka and Zlatko Pejić
info@makronova.com
www.makronova.com/posts.aspx?pageID=1

Christina Pirello
cp@christinacooks.com
www.christinacooks.com
www.christinapirello.org

Jessica Porter
www.hipchicksmacrobiotics.com/

Sheldon and Ginat Rice
shelgin@netvision.net.il
www.thericehouse.com/

Michael Rossoff
michael@michaelrossoff.com
www.michaelrossoff.com/

William Spear
www.williamspear.com
www.fortunateblessings.org

Bill Tara
www.billtara.net/

Francisco and Eugenia Varatojo
varatojo@e-macrobiotica.com
www.e-macrobiotica.com/

Verne Varona
vernevarona@earthlink.net
www.vernevarona.com/

Denny Waxman
dennywaxman@dennywaxman.com
http://strengthenhealth.org/index.php

INDEX

A

Abdominal breathing, 150–51

Abdominal chakra, 219

Acid-alkaline balance, 138, 177, 227–31. *See Also* Alkaline-forming diet

Acid mantle, 189

Acupressure points, 19, 115–18, 219–20, 256

Aihara, Cornelia, 260

Aihara, Herman, 3, 207, 227, 260

Alcohol, 18, 62, 122, 150, 228

Alkaline-forming diet, 287–89. *See Also* Acid-alkaline balance

Allergies, 187, 203

Almonds
    Orange Amasake Pudding, 327–28
    Rice Pudding, 309–10

Amasake Pudding, Orange, 327–28

Amino acids, 161

Antioxidants, 162

Apologizing, 44

Appetite, 134–35

Apples
    Fresh Golden Juice, 331
    Fresh Green Juice, 331
    Fresh Red Juice, 331
    Fried Apple Rings with Vanilla Pudding, 316

Red Quinoa, Tofu, and Vegetable Salad with Fresh Green Herbs and Egg, 298–99

Appreciation, 78–79, 259

Arame
    Red Quinoa, Tofu, and Vegetable Salad with Fresh Green Herbs and Egg, 298–99

Arthritis, 16, 203, 287

Ashburn, Leslie, 187

Asparagus, Corn, Tuna, Parsnip Fries, and Salad, 304–5

Associations, 115

Assumptions
    becoming habits, 35
    breaking free of, 35
    exercises on, 36–37
    giving meaning to, 32–33
    making, 32, 34, 51–52

Asthma, 287

Astrology, 251

Awareness
    of change, 210–11
    of eating, 225
    of emotions, 73–76, 94–95, 140
    of energy, 132–33, 225–26

B

Babies

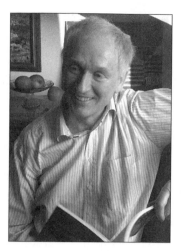

ABOUT THE AUTHOR

Best-selling author Simon Brown has been practicing a macrobiotic lifestyle for nearly thirty years. In the early1980s, he studied under leading macrobiotic experts Mishio and Aveline Kushi and Shizuko Yamamoto and, from 1986 to 1993, ran the Community Health Foundation in London, where he organized macrobiotic cooking classes, courses, and international seminars. This led to a successful career as a macrobiotic teacher and consultant.

Currently the chairperson of The Macrobiotic Association of Great Britain and the Feng Shui Society, the author also runs a thriving macrobiotic clinic that offers a range of courses and is part owner of a macrobiotic health food store and café. He is the author of *Modern-Day Macrobiotics* and has written several best-selling books on feng shui, face reading, and natural health. In addition, he is a highly regarded practitioner of shiatsu and a feng shui consultant who has advised thousands of individual clients as well as corporations like The Body Shop, British Airways, and various airports. Brown lives with his life partner, Dragana, and four sons in London, where he runs a popular international macrobiotic discussion group. For further information, visit www.chienergy.co.uk or contact him at simon@chienergy.co.uk.